ROUTLEDGE LIBRARY EDITIONS:
CHILDREN AND DISABILITY

Volume 12

T0372884

CARING FOR THE MENTALLY HANDICAPPED CHILD

CARING FOR THE MENTALLY HANDICAPPED CHILD

DAVID WILKIN

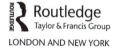
Routledge
Taylor & Francis Group

LONDON AND NEW YORK

First published in 1979 by Croom Helm Ltd

This edition first published in 2016
by Routledge
2 Park Square, Milton Park, Abingdon, Oxon OX14 4RN

and by Routledge
711 Third Avenue, New York, NY 10017

Routledge is an imprint of the Taylor & Francis Group, an informa business

British Library Cataloguing in Publication Data
A catalogue record for this book is available from the British Library

ISBN: 978-1-138-96230-9 (Set)
ISBN: 978-1-315-64761-6 (Set) (ebk)
ISBN: 978-1-138-12493-6 (Volume 12) (hbk)
ISBN: 978-1-315-64786-9 (Volume 12) (ebk)

Publisher's Note
The publisher has gone to great lengths to ensure the quality of this reprint but points out that some imperfections in the original copies may be apparent.

Disclaimer
The publisher has made every effort to trace copyright holders and would welcome correspondence from those they have been unable to trace.

The publishers would like to make it clear that the views and opinions expressed, and language used in the book are the author's own and a reflection of the times in which it was published. No offence is intended in this edition.

CARING FOR THE MENTALLY HANDICAPPED CHILD

DAVID WILKIN

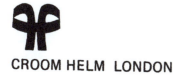

CROOM HELM LONDON

©1979 Crown
Croom Helm Ltd, 2-10 St John's Road, London SW11
ISBN 0-85664-648-2

British Library Cataloguing in Publication Data

Wilkin, David
    Caring for the mentally handicapped child.
    1. Mentally handicapped children – care and
    treatment – Great Britain
    I. Title
    362.7'8'30941   HV901.G7
    ISBN 0-85664-648-2

Printed in Great Britain by
Biddles Ltd, Guildford, Surrey

CONTENTS

PREFACE

The research on which this book is based was conducted for and funded by the Department of Health and Social Security between 1973 and 1976. It is now three years since the field work was completed. There have undoubtedly been some improvements in services for severely mentally handicapped children and their families in the intervening period, but these have not, unfortunately, removed some of the most pressing problems which beset mothers of such children. Whilst this book is often highly critical of those people who provide services to families it is recognised that they work under difficult conditions. They are constrained by a severe lack of resources and often by a lack of imaginative leadership from above. Changes in the knowledge and attitudes of those who actually provide services are necessary, but these will be ineffectual unless accompanied by increased resources, imaginative planning and effective leadership. I hope, therefore, that this book will be read by a wide audience, since it is addressed to anyone who is concerned for the welfare of the severely mentally handicapped and those who care for them.

The book is principally about mothers of severely mentally handicapped children rather than families or the children themselves. Community care of such children relies on the fact that these mothers are prepared to tolerate a burden which most people would consider intolerable. The study described here was only possible because the mothers were prepared to give up some of their valuable spare time to answer the questions put to them by myself and the other interviewers (Hilary Gellman, Joyce Goldstone and Cath Prior). I would like to express my thanks to them and I hope that the publication of the findings of this research will add some weight to efforts to obtain better services for them and for future generations of mothers of severely mentally handicapped children.

Whilst the views expressed in the following chapters are my own, I would like to thank Joyce Leeson and Karin Lowson for their hard work in providing many valuable comments, criticisms and suggestions at all stages of the preparation of the manuscript. I would also like to thank Professor Alwyn Smith who supervised the PhD thesis on which this book is based. Most books only reach completion through the goodwill and hard work of typists, and this is no exception. I am very grateful for the patience of Leila Britten who typed the manuscript and to Lee Skimore who typed the original thesis.

David Wilkin

September 1978

1 POLICIES FOR THE MENTALLY HANDICAPPED: PAST, PRESENT AND FUTURE

To many who are unfamiliar with the condition, the mentally handicapped are incomprehensible, at times frightening and usually best forgotten. To those who spend every day of their lives with a mentally handicapped person it is the attitudes of other people which are incomprehensible, at times frightening and usually best forgotten. Thousands of parents can describe the pleasures, as well as the trials and tribulations, of family life with a severely mentally handicapped person − to anyone who is prepared to listen and take an interest. It is unfortunate that even today many people know little about the mentally handicapped, although the last 50 years have seen some signs of progress in attitudes, at least in professional and governmental circles. It is no longer considered necessary that society should be protected from the mentally handicapped, but in spite of improvements in attitudes, and associated improvements in services, the mentally handicapped themselves and their families still face many problems. There is still a pressing need for increased understanding and for further improvements in attitudes and services beyond those that have already taken place.

This book is concerned with the problems experienced by families caring for children who were suffering from severe mental handicap, which has been described as 'a diverse condition which stems from an assortment of aetiological sources, covers a wide range of functional impairment and is attended by extremely varied social problems and issues'.[1] The only characteristic which is common to all people who are mentally handicapped is that they suffer varying degrees of mental impairment. Beyond this the differences between one mentally handicapped individual and another are often greater than the similarities. It is hardly surprising that a recent survey found that many people are unable to distinguish the mentally handicapped from the mentally ill, or to say what is meant by mental handicap.[2] Nevertheless, in virtually all societies, those who suffer from mental impairment are recognised as different in some way from other people, and in all advanced societies they are classified in separate legal and administrative categories. It is necessary therefore, at the outset, to devote some attention to the ways in which the mentally handicapped are identified and classified. Today

11

two main approaches to the definition of mental handicap can be distinguished; namely the medical/psychological approach and the sociological approach, and these will be briefly reviewed in this chapter. Following this the size of the problem, in terms of the numbers of mentally handicapped people will be considered. A number of studies in this country have estimated the prevalence of mental handicap and these will be briefly reviewed. Although this book focuses on the care and support provided by society for these people and their families, the present situation cannot be understood unless seen in historical perspective. Their present position is a product of the historical development of attitudes and services, and therefore this development will be summarised before briefly describing current government policies and the structure of the services. The chapter concludes with a discussion of some of the problems which will need to be overcome if society is to provide adequate services.

Definitions

The classifications and terminology used to define and refer to people with below average intellectual functioning have become increasingly complex as the need to classify and label has grown with the development of complex societies. The medical/psychological and sociological models constitute two fairly distinct approaches to the problem of defining the mentally handicapped and, although there is a considerable degree of overlap between them, their basic conceptions of the problem are different. Administrative and legal definitions do not constitute a separate approach; they are syntheses of the two basic models, sometimes drawing more on one and sometimes more on the other in different societies and during different historical periods.

The Medical/Psychological Model

The medical/psychological model makes use of a combination of pathological and statistical criteria to define mental handicap. Individuals are described and classified in terms of clinical abnormalities which are deemed to be responsible for a statistically low level of intellectual functioning. Within this general approach it is possible to make distinctions identifying separate medical, psychological and educational models, but for the purposes of this brief review they can be dealt with together, since they all adopt a supposedly 'objective' clinical view of the problem.[3] The helping professions (medicine, psychology, education, etc.) tend to define mental handicap in terms of 'the pattern of symptoms which characterises the condition and the operations which are used to determine whether these symptoms are present in an individual case'.[4]

Since significantly sub-average intellectual functioning is an essential component of this definition, the intelligence test has become the most widely used means of deciding whether any particular individual should be classified as mentally handicapped, retarded, subnormal, deficient, etc. Concern is mainly with the characteristics believed to be inherent in the individual, rather than with his or her social behaviour and the reaction of other people in the social environment. Thus it is possible for the clinician to diagnose mental handicap irrespective of whether or not any individual is identified by his or her social milieu as handicapped or abnormal. The combination of a distinct pathology and sub-average intellectual functioning determines the individual's assessment. Discrepancies between clinical assessments and the evaluation of lay people who come into contact with the handicapped person are rare in relation to the severely handicapped but are much more common in the case of mildly handicapped individuals.[5] The most widely accepted clinical definition is that proposed by the American Association for Mental Deficiency which states that: 'Mental retardation refers to sub-average general intellectual functioning which originates during the developmental period and is associated with impairment in adaptive behaviour.[6]

The other principle feature of the clinical view is the emphasis placed on the interdependence of mind and body. Intellectual deficiency is seen to be closely linked with physical deficiency. Thus Soddy, in a discussion of the medical approach to subnormality, says that ' . . . an inherent mental subnormality is more likely than not to be accompanied by a subnormality of body and vice versa'; and later: 'The inferiority of mind and body which is at the root of subnormality is usually reflected in individual appearance.'[7]

The Sociological Model

The other general approach to the definition of mental handicap is essentially sociological. Sociological concern with the problem of defining mental handicap stems from the observation that not all societies identify and label all individuals with sub-average intellectual functioning and impaired behaviour as a distinct group and, within societies in which people are so labelled, the application of the label sometimes seems arbitrary. The major differences between societies in classification and labelling mostly concern mildly handicapped individuals and seem to be related to differing levels of industrialisation. The proportion of the population reported to be mentally handicapped varies between 1 per cent and 16 per cent.[8] The most highly industrialised societies tend to report a higher proportion of mentally handicapped, reflecting the necessity for a relatively high level of intelligence in order to achieve 'social normality'. The sociologist is concerned with what factors are relevant in the selective application of the label within a group of people, all of whom may manifest similar objective behaviour. Why are individuals of similar intellectual ability classified as mentally handicapped in one society and normal in another? The answer to this question lies in an analysis of social roles. Society can be conceptualised as a network of interlocking social systems (e.g. family, neighbourhood, work, political party, sports club) in which each system consists of a group of statuses (e.g. mother, father, son, daughter in the family; or labourer, driver, clerk, foreman, manager at work). Each individual is a member of a number of different social systems with a certain status in each system dependent on factors such as age, sex, education, background, etc. For each status there is a set of prescribed behaviours which make up the role that a person is expected to play. Thus certain behaviour is expected of mothers, neighbours, mechanics, doctors, members of parliament, footballers, etc. The labelling of an individual as mentally handicapped is a response to his or her inability to conform to the role expectations of the usual statuses. Such a person is therefore granted an alternative and lower status, that of a mentally handicapped person, a role which he or she is able to fill. The ability to do intelligence tests and to reach a certain level of education is not, for most people in simple societies, a necessary prerequisite for adequate role performance, but the increasing social, political and industrial complexity of developed societies makes a certain minimum level of intelligence, education and training essential for most people. Thus it is not surprising that in developed societies far more individuals are identified as incompetent in the fulfilment of normal role expectations.[9]

The medical/psychological and sociological models do not, however, constitute simple alternatives and there are many variants within and overlapping them. The medical/psychological model, where it is used as a basis for professional practice, utilises implicit evaluations of social functioning, particularly at the borderlines between categories. For example, the DHSS Census of Mental Handicap Patients in Hospitals (1972) referred to the difficulty of classifying patients:

The level of mental development does not entirely determine

whether a patient is classified as subnormal or severely subnormal. Other items such as social competence are taken into account. The classification is thus, to some extent, a matter of judgement on the part of the clinician who assigns it.

Equally the sociological model is not applied in complete isolation from medical and psychological criteria, since those people clinically recognised as mentally handicapped, in a society where medicine is highly respected, are most likely to be those who are also socially recognised as mentally handicapped. The models which implicitly or explicitly are utilised by the professions working with the mentally handicapped (e.g. education, social work, nursing, etc.) tend to make use of both the medical/psychological model and the sociological model. Similarly, the current administrative/legal definition of mental handicap utilises both approaches.

The Administrative/Legal View

This has been subject to many changes historically which reflect changes in knowledge and a shifting balance of power between different professional groups. The historical development of official attitudes towards the mentally handicapped and the embodiment of these attitudes in legislation and administrative practices will be discussed later in this chapter. At present in Britain the legal definitions in the Mental Health Act of 1959 remain the basis for classification. The severely subnormal were said to possess:

> A state of arrested or incomplete development of mind which includes subnormality of intelligence and is of such a nature or degree that the patient is incapable of guarding himself against serious exploitation, or will be so incapable when of an age to do so.

The subnormal were distinguished from the severely subnormal principally on the basis of intelligence quotients, the dividing line being drawn at IQ 50. Supposedly objective measures of intelligence constitute the fundamental criterion for classification, but as noted above, these are tempered by a recognition of the importance of social competence in a reference to the ability of the patient to guard himself against serious exploitation. Although the terminology used has changed since 1959, the definition of mental handicap, and therefore the practice according to which individuals are classified, has remained the same.

The question of how borderline individuals come to be classified as either mildly or severely mentally handicapped is an important one, but cannot be pursued here. The research described in this book was concerned only with the experiences of families caring for an individual who had already been administratively labelled as severely mentally handicapped. Fortunately, from the point of view of the research, in most cases there tends to be little disagreement over the classification of an individual as severely handicapped. In the vast majority of those who are administratively so defined, a pathological condition, sub-average intellectual functioning and inability to fulfil normal role expectations are all apparent.

The Prevalence of Severe Mental Handicap

Given that there are variations between societies in the proportions of individuals classified as mentally handicapped, some information on the size of the problem according to the definition currently in use in this country is necessary. In considering the needs of mentally handicapped individuals and those caring for them, in terms of the services that might be provided, it is necessary to bear in mind the scale on which these provisions will be required. Precise assessments of the prevalence of severe mental handicap, as opposed to informed guesses, are difficult to come by for a number of reasons. Clearly the efficiency of assessment procedures, on which estimates of prevalence are based, can affect the accuracy of these estimates, and these procedures may vary considerably from one area to another. In addition, the accuracy of prevalence figures varies between different age groups. School-age children tend to be most readily identified, since there is a statutory requirement for education authorities to make special provision for all severely mentally handicapped children. The identification of pre-school children and adults is very much dependent upon the services available in a particular area, since where individuals are not in contact with the services it is likely that they will remain unrecognised. Thus estimates based on the total number of individuals known to the various services are likely to understate the size of the problem. The age group 15 to 19 years is therefore used as a basis for assessing total prevalence, since it is likely that virtually all individuals have been identified by this age and they are still in contact with the services. On the basis of a number of epidemiological studies, Kushlick estimated that 3.7 per 1,000 of the people who survive to the age of 15 to 19 are likely to be severely mentally handicapped.[10] Using these figures, the 1971 White Paper estimated that 'there are probably about 120,000 people in England and Wales who are severely mentally handicapped, of whom about

50,000 are children'.[11]

However, more recent evidence from mental handicap registers suggests that there are considerable fluctuations from time to time in the numbers of severely mentally handicapped. Fryers has reported recently that in Salford there was a considerable increase in the numbers of children during the 1960s, probably due to fewer dying in their early years, but this has been followed by a decline during the 1970s in line with the declining birth rate generally.[12] In the future, a combination of a rising birth rate and improved survival could once more result in a rapid increase in the numbers of severely mentally handicapped children. In terms of the total population of this country, the number of severely handicapped individuals seems relatively small, which may account to some extent for the reluctance of successive governments to identify this group as a major priority. However, if one considers that the total number of severely mentally handicapped people in this country is approximately the same as the population of a medium-sized town, it soon becomes apparent that providing the care, education and support that they and their families need is a major problem.

The Development of Official Attitudes

Although this book is concerned with families caring for severely mentally handicapped children in the 1970s, it is illuminating, from the point of view of understanding the problems and needs that they experience, to describe the historical development of attitudes and services. Current attitudes and services are the product of more than a century of change and development. The sort of services that families receive and the attitudes expressed by both lay and professional people are more easily understood when seen as part of a continuing process of development. The terminology used has changed a number of times over the years and, although in most of this book the term mental handicap is used, it is more appropriate when reviewing historical developments to make use of the different terms that have applied during different periods. Thus terms such as mental deficiency, feeble-mindedness, subnormality, etc. are used as appropriate.

Pre-twentieth Century

Even in the simplest of societies from the beginning of history there have probably been those who perceived that some of their fellow men were socially incompetent and very stupid, and reasoned that these factors were causally connected[13]

But the social recognition of these people as a distinct group, their administrative classification and their identification as a group deserving special attention is a much more recent phenomenon. An early land-mark was the publication, by Itard in 1801, of the pamphlet *L'Education du Sauvage D'Aveyron*, followed in 1828 by the setting up of the first institute for the education and training of the mentally defective in Paris. Nineteenth-century developments in medical science and education for the masses, which were closely associated with rapid industrial development in most European countries, meant that for the first time it was felt necessary to attempt to classify, treat and educate the mentally handicapped as a special group. Development in England was slow in comparison to most European countries and, although some attempts were made to treat idiots separately, the 1890 Lunacy Act made no distinction between idiots (the mentally handicapped) and persons of unsound mind (the mentally ill).[14]

To the extent that the mentally handicapped were separately iden-tified and treated in nineteenth-century England, this was usually in the context of the disease model, which sought to establish 'causes' and appropriate measures of treatment which would result in cures, or at least prevention. However, the failure to account for mental deficiency in terms of pathological conditions with known causes, and the apparent hopelessness of attempts at treatment, resulted in a marked loss of interest in the problems of this group by medical practitioners. As far as education was concerned, the development of elementary education for all children following the 1870 Education Act was such an enormous task that there was a tendency to lose sight of the needs of special groups such as the mentally handicapped. Thus only 3 per cent of more than 29,000 idiots in institutions in 1881 were receiving care and treat-ment in institutions designed for them.[15] The failure of medicine to identify causes and develop treatments led, in the early twentieth century, to a marked shift in the type of explanations offered for the condition. Where causes were not obvious and treatments were not available it became fashionable to resort to moralistic explanations. Fernald in 1912 summed up this attitude to the high grade or feeble-minded:

> The feeble-minded are a parasitic, predatory class, never capable of self support or of managing their own affairs ... they cause unutter-able sorrow at home and are a menace and danger to the community. The feeble minded are almost invariably immoral, and if at large usually become carriers of venereal disease or give birth to children

who are as defective as themselves. The feeble minded woman who marries is twice as prolific as the normal woman.

Every feeble minded person, especially the high grade imbecile, is a potential criminal, needing only the proper environment and opportunity for the development and expression of his criminal tendencies. The unrecognised imbecile is a most dangerous element in the community.[16]

The 1913 Mental Deficiency Act

Associated with the growth of moralistic explanations was the development of genetic theories. Put in their crudest form, these theories suggested that, since handicapping conditions were inherited, they could be eliminated by preventing carriers or sufferers from breeding. These developments resulted in a growing public awareness of, and interest in, the subject of mental deficiency during the early years of the century, which led to the appointment of a Royal Commission on the care of the feeble minded in 1904. Although the Commission reported in 1908, the government did not introduce a Bill into Parliament until 1912. The resulting Act of 1913 was largely based on the recommendations of the Royal Commission.

Jones, in her excellent history of the mental health services, noted that the Act made possible a rapid development in provision for defectives and, in spite of the predominantly medical and educational influences which had shaped it, dealt with mental deficiency in an adult primarily in social terms.[17] The effect of the Act was to place mental handicap in a socio-legal framework, but the main emphasis was on providing custodial care and protecting other members of the community, rather than on providing education, care, treatment and support for the mentally handicapped. The custodial nature of the Act was reflected in the fact that the Boards of Control which were established were quite separate from the Ministry of Health, and Local Authority Mental Deficiency Committees were responsible to the officers of the Clerks of the Councils rather than to health departments. Jaehnig has pointed out that the prevailing moralistic ideology in the early years of the century provided a powerful cause for the establishment of institutions to control the mentally deficient, keep the sexes apart and keep them all out of sight.[18] Hollander writing in 1916 summed up this attitude:

Idiots should never be kept at home, but sent to special homes for permanent care. Parents must realise that though such children can never be brought up to be normal, they can be considerably improved, mentally and physically if trained at an early age by competent teachers.[19]

One of the most important features of the 1913 Act was the requirement on Local Authorities to identify mental defectives resident in their administrative area and to assume supervision of those identified. When the Act came into force the number of known defectives bore no real relationship to the number requiring treatment. By 1920, 10,129 defectives had been identified, but this was still only a small proportion of the whole, and by 1927 the number had risen to well over 60,000.[20] The emphasis in the Act on ascertaining, controlling, segregating and supervising mental defectives was becoming apparent in practice. This was hardly surprising given the administrative legal nature of the provisions and the bodies set up to implement them. During this period doctors probably spent more time identifying and classifying mental defectives than they spent in treating them. However, by the late 1920s the Board of Control began to realise the impossibility of providing institutional facilities for all mental defectives.

At first, community care was only seen as a rather unsatisfactory expedient. Shrubshall and Williams stated very tentatively in 1932 that 'under favourable circumstances a defective might be kept at home'.[21] The first signs of a major change in prevailing attitudes came with the report of the Wood Committee in 1929. The Committee's report marked a considerable step forward in that it recommended a social definition of deficiency, greater use of all forms of community care and a co-ordinated mental health service. However, although the report resulted in a considerable development of community facilities, its recommendations were not to be implemented fully for many years and moralistic views remained much in evidence. Statutory supervision of the mentally deficient often amounted to surveillance and stress was laid on the adequacy of parents in caring for the defective person. But the moralistic ideology was not the only reason for the failure to develop community care. The economic climate of the 1930s was not conducive to integrating the mentally handicapped in the community. The economic situation did not encourage authorities to spend money on the provision of community services and many families, who might otherwise have wished to keep a handicapped person at home, found that it was financially advantageous to them if he or she was admitted to institutional care. Parents managing on unemployment benefit simply could not afford the additional expense involved in caring for a severely handicapped child.

The Post-war Period

In spite of the emphasis placed on providing institutional facilities there was never really any prospect of providing a sufficient number of places to cater for all severely mentally handicapped people. Indeed it was more or less inevitable that the majority would continue to be cared for by their families. Not surprisingly, therefore, the attention of professional groups concerned with their care and treatment began to shift to the family in the post-war period. The child guidance movement, which was imported from the USA in the 1930s, and the post-war development of psychotherapy emphasised the importance of viewing the abnormal individual in his natural environment, the family, and of viewing the whole family as the patient. During the 1950s the views of Bowlby became very influential in moulding the attitudes of the professions dealing with the mentally handicapped in the community. The maintenance of the maternal affectional bond came to be seen as imperative, almost at any cost.[22] Although many people felt that the presence of a mentally handicapped person had harmful psychological, emotional and social effects on the family, the necessity of developing community mental health services rather than concentrating efforts on the provision of institutional care was becoming more widely accepted. The provisions of the 1913 Act came under critical review with the establishment of the Royal Commission on the Law Relating to Mental Illness and Mental Deficiency in 1954. The Commission recommended a shift in emphasis from hospital care to community responsibility for both the mentally ill and the mentally handicapped. Their report contained the basic elements of a comprehensive family-oriented system of community care: thus residential or hospital care was seen as appropriate only where the burdens placed on the family were too great or where special circumstances existed.

The 1959 Mental Health Act

The basic principles of the Commission's report were embodied in the Act of 1959. It contained a new orientation to the definition of mental handicap. The terms idiot, imbecile and feeble-minded were replaced by severely subnormal and subnormal, the definitions of which were essentially sociological with no clear lines of division drawn. The severely subnormal were distinguished from the subnormal on the grounds that they were incapable of leading an independent life or of guarding against serious exploitation. In terms of care and treatment, emphasis was laid on the development of community facilities and the care of the subnormal person in the family. It was envisaged that the majority of the mentally handicapped would be cared for in their own family homes except in certain specific circumstances, and that local health and welfare authorities would be responsible for providing the advice, support, training facilities and other services required by families. However, although some of the services were made obligatory for local authorities, others, such as welfare services in the home and the provision of residential homes and hostels, remained permissive powers. For the majority of families the Act did not produce any immediate improvement in their conditions, but its basic orientation did lead to changes in the degree of involvement of different professional groups dealing with the mentally handicapped. Psychologists, social workers, teachers, speech therapists gradually gained in stature whilst traditional medical involvement declined. The social competence of the handicapped person and the psychological and emotional competence of the parents became the principal foci of professional attention.

Titmuss pointed out in 1961 that community care was not a new concept. The 1951 McIntosh Report on social workers in the mental health service had advocated the development of such a policy. He commented:

> What progress have we made since 1951 in working out, in terms of the medical, psychological, social and economic needs of the individual, the concept of community care? . . . beyond a few brave ventures . . . one cannot find much evidence of attempts to hammer out the practice, as distinct from the theory, of community care for the mentally ill and subnormal.[23]

Certainly the 1959 Act did not spell out in facts and figures how such a service would be developed, but in 1963 the government issued a document entitled *The Development of Community Care* which outlined local authority plans for the next decade.[24] The services recommended were family oriented:

> It is usually best for the mentally disordered person in the community, whether adult or child, to live at home where this is possible . . . the services provided inside and outside the home can improve an unfavourable situation and make it unnecessary to seek an alternative.[25]

The sentiments sounded fine, but the details of the plans and the facts and figures on which they were based left a lot to be desired.

Although it espoused the principles of community care, the document
went on to suggest that more mentally handicapped individuals might
require residential care. The provisions proposed for community
services (numbers of training centre places, health visitors, home helps,
home nurses and social workers) were not an adequate basis for comprehensive care. Nevertheless, they were sufficient to show that most
local authorities were not adequately prepared to assume responsibility
for community care and that there were enormous disparities in the
levels of provision provided in different areas. The document was
described as 'one of the most disappointing publications in the mental
health field for many years'.[26] The remainder of the 1960s did not see
the flowering of what Titmuss described as the everlasting cottage
garden trailer: community care. The Seebohm Report in 1968 stated
that: 'The widespread belief that we have community care of the
mentally disordered is, for many parts of the country, still a sad illusion
and judging by published plans will remain so for many years ahead.'[27]
However, as Jaehnig has pointed out, the Seebohm Committee itself did
little to remedy this situation. It made no attempt to describe what
would constitute an effective family service although it made frequent
reference to such a service.[28]

In summary then, the 1959 Act marked a significant shift in the
orientation of stated policy, from the provision of institutional care to a
system of family-based community care, but the reality for the majority
of families hardly changed. Perhaps the most significant change
which followed the Act was the increased involvement of new professions, although it is debatable whether the advance of social work,
teaching and psychology made much difference to the lives of the
mentally handicapped and their families. Progress seemed to be painfully slow, but in 1967 the subject of the mentally handicapped came
sharply back into the news. Publication of allegations of staff cruelty
and misconduct at the Ely Hospital in Cardiff and Farleigh Hospital in
Somerset, and the enquiries set up by the DHSS to look into these
allegations, raised many questions.[29] It appeared to most observers that,
as well as failing to create adequate community services, the government
had also failed to ensure that conditions in hospitals were improved.
Two years later, Pauline Morris's book *Put Away* was published.[30] It
helped to stimulate a growing demand for a thorough review of all the
services for the mentally handicapped and put forward concrete proposals for the reorganisation of hospitals.

Better Services for the Mentally Handicapped

In June 1971 the government published its White Paper, *Better Services for the Mentally Handicapped*, which still provides the main guidelines for the provision of services. The terms subnormal and severely subnormal were discarded in favour of mentally handicapped and severely mentally handicapped, in order to;

> . . . emphasise that our attitude should be the same as to other types of handicap, i.e. to prevent it whenever possible, to assess it adequately when it occurs, and to do everything possible to alleviate its severity and compensate for its effects.[31]

The general principles put forward in the White Paper did not differ markedly from those contained in the Mental Health Act twelve years earlier. Family-oriented community care was the central theme: 'Each handicapped person should live with his own family as long as this does not impose an undue strain on them or him, and he and his family should receive full advice and support.'[32]

The White Paper provided substantial lists of services and assistance needed by the mentally handicapped and their families, but when it came to a discussion of actual provisions, the promises contained in the general principles were not fulfilled. The emphasis on family-based services carried less conviction when it was noted that the government was actually forecasting a 15 per cent increase in the number of mentally handicapped people in residential care.[33] As far as domiciliary services were concerned, the White Paper failed to describe in any detail what the government considered would constitute an effective service. In addition to this, no planning targets for domiciliary services were produced, on the grounds that it would be extremely difficult to do so because such services cover a number of different client groups other than the mentally handicapped. This failure to stipulate the necessary details of the services required removed some of the credibility that statements of general principle might otherwise have had.

Despite the inadequacies of the White Paper, services for the mentally handicapped and their families have made some progress since 1971. In the period in which it was introduced (1969/70 to 1972/73) the growth of revenue expenditure on mental handicap services was more than double the growth rate in real terms for the health and personal social services overall.[34] Additional expenditure has continued to be directed towards services for this group, but much of this increased expenditure has been on residential facilities, upgrading hospital accommodation and providing additional education and training facilities. Improvements in the sometimes appalling conditions which existed in the hospitals prior to 1971 were absolutely essential and, in line with the government's intention to provide more locally-based residential accommodation and less accommodation in the large hospitals, it was equally important to allocate resources to the provision of alternative residential accommodation. Similarly, there was a need for improvements in education and training. The transfer of responsibility for the education of the mentally handicapped from local health authorities to education authorities, in the same year as the White Paper was produced, has resulted in considerable improvements in the facilities for schooling many severely handicapped children. There have also been increases in the number of training centre places available for adults. However, in spite of the additional resources which have been provided for these services, there is still considerable scope for further improvement. There are many mentally handicapped people, including children, still cared for in hospitals who do not require and probably do not benefit from this sort of care, and there remain some hospitals where the facilities and standards of care leave much to be desired. Whilst most mentally handicapped children are now able to attend school, there is still a grave shortage of training centre places for adults in many areas. Jones, in a study carried out in 1974, found that local authority plans for education, training centre and residential provisions for the next ten years were already falling short of the guidelines laid down in the White Paper. She found a tendency to look for cheap solutions rather than solutions which would involve a real assumption of extra responsibility.[35]

Whilst education, training, hospital and residential facilities have seen some improvements since 1971, domiciliary services, unfortunately, seem to have remained more or less static. The policies of successive governments towards services for the mentally handicapped reflect an over-emphasis on institutional provisions. The emphasis has been on hospitals, residential units, training centres and schools, rather than on employing qualified people with resources at their disposal to provide support for the families who have undertaken the burden of caring for the majority of severely mentally handicapped individuals. Attitudes towards the care of the mentally handicapped have changed, but the residues of the philosophy that produced the 1913 Mental Deficiency Act are still influential. To what extent can we say that the principle of a comprehensive family-based service has been implemented? The only major development since 1971, in terms of direct support to families, has been the introduction of the Constant Attendance Allowance under the Chronically Sick and Disabled Persons Act of 1970. Most families have found that the allowance has done much to alleviate their financial difficulties, although many have had difficulty in obtaining it. However, little has been done to alleviate the many other problems which families experience. The reorganisation of social services that followed the Seebohm Report in 1968 has not, in general, greatly benefited the mentally handicapped and may have led to a deterioration in some areas. Jones commented that:

> Work with the mentally handicapped forms only a small part of the total responsibilities now facing social services departments; and the present emphasis on genericism in social work has created a certain resistance to planning for special groups. But the problems of this group are acute and likely to become more so.[36]

Problems for the Present and the Future

> The problems faced by parents of severely handicapped children in our society are at once so immediately demanding and so unremittingly persistent that they embarrass the imagination of those who have been spared them ... The mentally handicapped ... offend public taste by drawing attention to aspects of the human condition which our society finds unmentionable.[37]

In spite of official statements about integrating the mentally handicapped into the community at large, the problems that the Newsons referred to above still exist both among lay people and among those responsible for the care and treatment of the mentally handicapped. The birth of such a child is regarded by society as a tragic event which has damaging consequences for individuals and the family unit. It creates a handicapped family. The Newsons go on to say: 'So society piles on the final indignity by suggesting parents of handicapped children are no longer capable of making rational judgements about what is best either for their own children or for themselves.[38] It is these attitudes which underlie the failure to implement policies designed to create services which support the family as the basic unit of care.

Whilst existing services leave much to be desired, there are grounds for cautious optimism with regard to the future. There is considerable pressure for change from many sources, and detailed proposals for the development of effective services have been formulated. Where these have been implemented, even on a limited scale, the results have been encouraging. A number of voluntary and professional organisations have, since the White Paper was issued, produced the sort of guidelines for the development of family-oriented services which were lacking in the White Paper.[39] There remains a gulf between such proposals and their implementation in the form of services, although there are signs that real efforts are being made at local and national level to evaluate services currently available, to lay down specific plans for the improvement of services and to seek new solutions to the practical problems faced by families. The National Development Group, appointed by Barbara Castle in 1976, has played an important role in this process. In its advice to authorities responsible for the provision of services it has concentrated on offering practical solutions to practical problems.[40] Over the past two years government committees have reported on the future of child health services and education facilities for the handicapped, and the report of the Committee on Mental Handicap Nursing is expected in the near future.[41] Despite many short-comings, these documents mark a considerable step forward in that attempts are being made to specify the content of comprehensive family-oriented services. It remains to be seen, however, whether the resources will be made available to implement these proposals nationally.

The desirability of particular policies and whether or not they can be implemented must not be judged in isolation from much wider economic and social issues. Services for the mentally handicapped have suffered and will continue to suffer as a consequence of the economic position of the country and the policies adopted to deal with the problems. Economic constraints have held back the development of health and social services as a whole, but powerless client groups such as the mentally handicapped, the mentally ill and the elderly are particularly vulnerable in the face of such constraints. Some commentators have argued that these constraints provide a stimulus for re-evaluation of services, or that they can be used to justify community services against residential services on the grounds that the former are cheaper. Whilst re-evaluation of services and reassessment of priorities is necessary, it is misleading to argue that a curtailment of public expenditure is compatible with the creation of a better service for the mentally handi-capped and their families. Good community services will almost cer-tainly cost a great deal of money and we should beware of attempts to sell the idea of community care on the grounds of cheapness. A cheap system of community care is likely to be one which exploits the families of the mentally handicapped. It can only be hoped that the economic situation improves and that, in the context of such an improvement, services for the mentally handicapped receive a satisfactory priority.

Economic constraints upon services may or may not be temporary in nature, but the care of the mentally handicapped always takes place in a given social context and the effects of social change may have profound implications for that care. The planning of services must include an awareness of current social trends and the likely directions of social change in the next few decades. Certain assumptions about the community and the family are usually implicit in official statements about the care of the mentally handicapped. They are based on models which are rarely made explicit and which are also usually static, and therefore fail to take account of changes in family structure and the attitudes and expectations of the individuals who comprise families. Community care rests very heavily on the family, and family care rests equally heavily on assumptions about the role of women in the home and in society at large; assumptions which may no longer be valid. The past 20 years have seen gradual changes taking place in the position of women in society. In particular, the number of women in employment outside the home has increased rapidly, and more recently we have seen changes in the social and legal status of women. However, for the majority of women, sharp contradictions exist between their position in society at large and their position at home. The domestic division of labour has remained relatively unchanged in spite of changes taking place outside the home. For mothers of severely mentally handicapped children such contradictions are particularly sharp. The daily routine of child care and housework for such mothers becomes a daily grind which effectively prevents most of them from playing a full role in life outside the home. It is unlikely that these mothers will continue to accept such a situation indefinitely. Outside the family, community care rests on an implicit model of community which takes little account of changes in housing, transport, communications, etc. Families are assumed to have close supportive networks of relatives and friends who are able to lend a hand, and to live amongst neighbours whom they can call on to help out at a moment's notice. The reality is often very different. For families with a severely mentally handicapped member, the need for such support has remained whilst potential sources of support have tended to dwindle. In theory these informal sources have been replaced by the services provided by the welfare state, but to what extent do services for the mentally handicapped and their families really provide support for the day-to-day domestic tasks which constitute the reality of community care? Subsequent chapters in this book will describe the realities of life for families who are caring for a severely mentally handicapped child. They will suggest in what ways services need to be improved to take account of the changing needs and expectations of families and of the individuals that carry the burden of care.

2 THE FAMILY AND THE HANDICAPPED PERSON

The gradual development of the view that the best place for the care of the severely mentally handicapped person is in his or her family home was in part a response to the realisation that providing institutional care for all severely mentally handicapped people would be very costly. It seemed unlikely that sufficient resources would ever be made available to provide good residential facilities. There was also, however, a growing campaign asserting the effects of home care as compared with institutional care on both normal and handicapped children. Bowlby, in the early 1950s, summarised studies of children in institutions as compared to those living at home and attributed the slower rate of development among the former to the absence of maternal affectional bonds.[1] Although much of Bowlby's thesis has since been challenged, his arguments were welcomed by those who argued for a reduction in institutional facilities and for more emphasis on family support services.

By the 1960s evidence was accumulating which clearly showed that severely mentally handicapped children raised in small family-like settings made more progress and presented fewer behaviour problems than those living in large wards in institutions.[2] The presentation of research findings which advocated family care rather than institutional care coincided with a marked shift in official policies in line with the 1959 Mental Health Act, which emphasised the importance of community services for the mentally handicapped and their families. Such policies were based largely on the documented disadvantages of institutional care; relatively little was known about the implications of the alternative, home care. It became necessary to ask, what are the practical psychological and emotional effects on the family? How much support does the family receive from the community and from the services? Why do some families seek long-term institutional care for their handicapped member whilst others do not? Considerable attention has therefore been devoted to seeking the answers to these and related questions during the last 20 years. This chapter will examine recent literature on families with a mentally handicapped member. First, general approaches to the problems will be considered, identifying two basic orientations. These will be followed by a discussion of psychological, social and practical problems experienced by families as a whole and by individual family members. The relationship between the family and the community will then be considered in terms of the availability of support from both formal sources (services) and informal sources (relatives, friends and neighbours). Finally, factors related to the admission of the handicapped person to long-term institutional care will be examined.

Two Contrasting Approaches to the Problem

There seem to be two basic professional and research orientations to the care of the handicapped person in the family, those based on a 'pathological' model and those based on a 'normal' family model. These start from fundamentally different assumptions concerning the impact of the handicapped person on family life, and therefore lead to an emphasis on different aspects of family organisation and functioning. Clearly the birth of a handicapped child has important long-term implications for the family. His or her presence is likely to slow down the gradual progress through the cycle of family life, and ultimately to result in its arrest. Instead of the parents eventually losing the responsibility for child care as their children grow up and leave home, they are faced with an indefinite period with a dependent child. More immediately, the family is faced with a burden, in terms of care and management, which is beyond their expectations of 'normal' children. However, what questions are asked about this situation and what answers are obtained largely depend on which of the two models mentioned above is adopted as a framework for viewing the problem.

Many writers have taken as self-evident the proposition that the birth and presence of a handicapped child will have damaging effects on the family as a unit and upon the individuals within it. Dupont, at a symposium on severely mentally retarded children living at home said: 'The development of a family life of near normal character, not only for the parents but also for the other siblings, is beyond the possibilities for most of these parents.'[3] The birth of the handicapped child is seen as a tragic event in the life of the family, the consequences being analogous to the consequences for the individual of the onset of an incurable disease. Kew, in a study of the siblings of handicapped children, after defining the family with a handicapped child as a handicapped family, goes on to say: 'The handicapped family faces certain special problems which actively disrupt the normal functioning of the family and often demand a readjustment of role relationships among its members.'[4] However, no attempt is usually made by the authors of this type of approach to say what they mean by the concept of 'normal family'. One suspects that, even if it were possible to arrive at an agreed

definition of what constitutes a normal family, it would either exclude
a large proportion of families or be so vague as to be virtually meaningless. Depending on the definition, large families, small families, one-
parent families, poor families, rich families, extended families, immi-
grant families, rural families, inner-city families and a host of others
might all be regarded as abnormal.

This pathological model still underlies much professional thinking
about the treatment, care and support of the mentally handicapped
individual and his or her family. The tendency of professionals to
advocate institutional care for the handicapped child, reported by both
Hewett and Jaehnig, is a reflection of this approach in professional
practice.[5] There is, unfortunately, much research literature which seems
to justify this approach, examples of which will be discussed later.
Many of the research findings leave much to be desired from a
methodological viewpoint, but the fundamental problem inherent in
the approach lies in its initial assumptions concerning the impact of the
child on the family. The behaviour of families is interpreted as abnormal
whatever they do. Jaehnig sums up the dilemma that families are faced
with as a consequence of the application of the pathological model in
professional practice:

> If they seek to contain his condition within the home they are open
> to accusations of being over-protective and retarding the child's
> further development. If they try to maintain a normal pattern of
> living inside and outside the home, they are failing to 'accept' the
> child's handicap, seen as another sign of emotional maladjustment.
> If they admit their child to residential care they encounter social
> disapproval for rejecting him and feel a need to justify their actions
> to others.[6]

The other main approach to the family with a handicapped member
emphasises the essential normality of the family and takes parental
statements about the nature of their situation at face value. When
parents say 'We are just like any other family', this is not interpreted as
an attempt to deny or conceal reality but as an expression of a perfectly legitimate view of their situation. The independent significance of
the parents' own interpretations of their circumstances is emphasised,
rather than professional interpretations which tend to apply external
criteria of normality. Whilst it is recognised that families with a handicapped member are subject to strains and stresses, it is pointed out that
a handicapped child is just as likely as any other child to be born into a

family with pre-existing strains and stresses. Hewett emphasised the 'normality' of many of the problems experienced by families with a handicapped child and concluded that such families 'meet the day to day problems that handicap creates with patterns of behaviour that, in many respects, deviate little from the norms derived from studying the families of normal children. They have more similarities with ordinary families than differences from them.'[7]

The process of defining the situation in which a family with a handicapped member finds itself extends also the child himself. Jaehnig found that the parents he interviewed emphasised the child's normality and resemblance to non-handicapped children. He emphasised that most of the parents described their child as a 'child with a handicap' rather than a 'handicapped child'.[8] The distinction is important because, in the former term, the emphasis is on the fact that he is a child, whereas in the latter the emphasis is on the handicap. Voysey takes the discussion of normality and implied abnormality further by looking at the reasons why parents of mentally handicapped children invoke normality in statements concerning the child. She maintains that such statements can be seen as attempts to appear to conform to the official norms and values of society regarding the family, and that the image of the family contained in official morality does not reflect reality for a majority of families, but is rather something which people attempt to subscribe to by the way in which they present their situation to others.[9] Thus, when the family with a mentally handicapped member describes itself as normal, it is only doing the same as most ordinary families, which also present themselves as conforming to the official morality.

To summarise, where the normal family model is used, the fact that problems are experienced by the family is not denied, but the assumption that one should always look for harmful effects is questioned. Consequently, the type of problems identified and the ways in which they are dealt with differ from those identified when the pathological model is used. Adopting an approach which has its origins in a pathological model Margaret Adams offers some advice to social workers:

> Because of the great practical difficulties associated with mental defect the social worker is frequently tempted into offering help and though this may often serve a useful ancillary purpose in temporarily relieving some minor pressure, she must remember that the emotional burden is not affected, and, in some cases, material help inappropriately offered may be something of an irritant because it

does not touch on the real issue of the emotional stress.[10]

In contrast Jaehnig, viewing families with a handicapped child as essentially normal, says:

> The focus of attention is drawn by the problems of practical management encountered by parents rather than the disturbance of interpersonal relations suggested by professional models pertaining to the families of the mentally handicapped to be their main problems.[11]

Effects on the Family

The impact that the handicapped person has on various aspects of family life has attracted much attention over the past 20 years. The way in which this subject has been dealt with and the particular focus of interest has varied greatly and has been much influenced by whether the problems were approached within the framework of the pathological model or the normal family model. Where the former has been the starting point it has resulted in a tendency to over-emphasise the psychological effects on the family, whilst authors who have viewed the family with a handicapped member as essentially normal have tended to stress the practical and material problems experienced.

Psychological Effects

References to the psychologically damaging effect of the handicapped person on other family members abound in the literature. Reactions of guilt, over-protection, rejection and non-acceptance are predicted for parents. Holt, in a study of the effects of a severely mentally handicapped child on the family, considered that 'the emotions of guilt and shame were very noticeable in most parents', although how these emotions were defined or measured is not clear.[12] One suspects that such statements were simply based on the author's impressions which, in the light of the fact that professional models tend to predict that such emotions will be felt, is not a very reliable source of information. Despite the fact that many people have expressed a need for caution in the use of such words as 'rejected'; this and other related terms are still commonly used both in professional literature and practice.[13] So common was the view that parents would exhibit feelings of rejection, guilt, shame, etc., that one author said that when he began working as a psychiatrist in subnormality, he sat back and waited for the hordes of guilty and aggressive parents to descend on him, but after eight long years he was still waiting for them in 1963.[14]

Where attempts have been made to measure emotional responses to the handicapped family member they have largely depended either on subjective evaluations by third parties or the use of attitude inventories or questionnaires, which are difficult to interpret because of limited information about 'normal' responses.[15] In spite of the lack of clear evidence, assumptions about the impact of the handicapped child on the psychological state of the parents still persist. For example McMichael, studying families with disabled children, devoted much attention to scoring the amount of 'rejection', 'over-anxiety' and 'over-protection' of their child shown in parents' responses. However, she provided no satisfactory definition of these terms, and the methods of measurement left a lot to be desired. The measure of 'rejection' was based on the frequency of contact with the teacher and the level of interest in the child's progress at school, a low level of contact and lack of interest being interpreted as 'rejection'.[16] It would be difficult to devise a more culturally biased means of assessing rejection. If these behaviours signify rejection, then very large numbers of parents who display no interest in their children's progress at school, perhaps because they do not attach any great importance to educational achievement or because they expect little success, must be described as rejecting parents. Another writer, Ronald MacKeith, a paediatrician writing in 1973, referred to parental feelings of revulsion, inadequacy, anger, grief, shock, guilt, bereavement and embarrassment.[17] Wolfensberger, however, pointed out that, to the extent that such feelings do exist among parents with a mentally handicapped child, they are probably perfectly normal responses and do not warrant the attention that has been devoted to them.[18] Most parents achieve a satisfactory adjustment to the psychological and emotional problems in a remarkably short space of time, as is evidenced by the large numbers of families who never seek or receive the 'support' of professional workers who would identify and help them over their 'abnormal' responses. Gath, in a study of families caring for a child with Down's Syndrome, reported that most families suffered some degree of stress but concluded:

Despite the understandable emotional reaction to the fact of the baby's abnormality, most of the families in this study have adjusted well and two years later are providing a home environment that is stable and enriching for both their normal and handicapped children. The findings of this study should not be interpreted as meaning that all parents with a child with a congenital malformation need either a marriage guidance counsellor or a psychiatrist.[19]

It is the practical and material difficulties of caring for a severely handicapped child that take much longer to come to terms with and with which many parents would welcome professional help.

One might expect that, if the psychological disruption created by the handicapped child is as great as is often suggested, this would result in a higher than average reported level of psychiatric symptoms among parents. Wing reported that, although 40 per cent of mothers of severely mentally handicapped children reported current psychiatric symptoms and 17 per cent had received treatment in the previous year, the figures were very similar to those found for women in the general population by Hare and Shaw and by Shepherd *et al.*[20] Most of the mothers interviewed by Wing, however, did attribute their symptoms to the presence of the handicapped child. Such a finding is hardly surprising though, since the handicapped child is clearly a source of considerable strain on many others, as will be evident later in this book. Parents of mentally handicapped children respond to stress in much the same way as any other parents and, in individual cases, the problems associated with such a child can place a severe strain on the mental health of the parents. Recognising this is, however, completely different from the assumption that all parents of handicapped children suffer psychological and emotional damage for which they require the services of doctors and social workers.

Although most attention has been directed towards the psychological adjustment of the parents, the siblings of the handicapped child have also been studied. Since the psycho-therapeutic model stresses the importance of viewing the whole family as the patient, adverse responses among siblings would be predicted. The problems of measuring siblings' emotional adjustment are exactly the same as those described above for parents. Two American studies, Farber in 1959 and Fowle in 1968, have reported that siblings' emotional adjustment was likely to be affected by the presence of a handicapped child, but the majority of studies which have looked at the adjustment of siblings have not provided much support for this view.[21] In spite of the contradictory evidence from research findings, the notion that most, if not all, siblings will be adversely affected is still given credence, especially among doctors. Such beliefs apparently find support in a recent study in this country of the siblings of handicapped children which found considerable problems of adjustment. However, the sample was selected from the records of a social work agency and the results were based on social workers' assessments of the family situation.[22] The fact that the families were already in contact with a social work agency indicates that either the parents or the professionals involved considered that they had problems which were amenable to social work intervention; thus the families were unlikely to be representative of all families with a handicapped child. In addition, the emphasis in much social work training on the psychologically damaging impact of the handicapped child on family members may well have influenced the social workers' assessments of siblings' adjustment. In another study, parents frequently stated that siblings had suffered adverse effects, although they were not asked for details of these effects. Undoubtedly the presence of a handicapped brother or sister must have some effects on their lives, but whilst these may be psychologically or emotionally damaging this is not necessarily the case. It might, perhaps, advance our understanding a great deal more to ask the siblings themselves what they feel has been the effect of living with a handicapped child. Personal observation indicates that many would point to the beneficial, as well as the adverse effects, as do their parents. A study which interviewed older siblings of handicapped children in New York found 'a surprising number of brothers and sisters of retarded children who appeared to us to have benefitted in some way from the experiences of growing up with a handicapped sibling'.[23]

Social Effects

Social effects can be divided into those concerned with relationships within the family and those concerned with the relationship between the family and the outside social world. One of the most comprehensive studies of the effects of a handicapped child on relationships between parents was carried out by Farber in 1959. He looked at the degree of marital integration (i.e. the stability and cohesiveness of the marriage) in 175 families where the child was living at home and 65 in which the child had been admitted to an institution. He found a higher level of integration among parents of mentally retarded girls than boys and noted that placing the child in an institution improved marital integration. The degree of dependence of the handicapped child did not appear to affect marital integration but was shown to have an adverse effect on siblings.[24] However, as in the case of the evidence of psychologically damaging effects, criticisms can be made of the methods of assessment used, and there is sufficient conflicting evidence to throw doubts on Farber's findings. Carr has pointed out that Farber's concept of marital integration is based on parents having similar attitudes and behaviour, thus assuming low integration in the many successful marriages in which the partners possess qualities and interests very different from each other but in which there is no conflict because the qualities and interests are complementary.[25] Conflicting evidence also came from Tizard and Grad's study of families, which concluded that keeping the handicapped child at home could not be shown to have adverse effects on family life.[26] More recently, Fowle conducted a similar study to Farber's and found no difference in marital integration between families with male and female retardates and between those whose child was at home and those whose child was in an institution.[27]

The social impact of the handicapped person in terms of producing an arrest in the family cycle has already been mentioned at the beginning of this chapter. Schild has argued that this arrest in the family cycle, caused by the long-term dependency of the handicapped child, produces role tensions within the family, and that all family members have to undergo a process of redefining their roles as family members. For example, the parents are forced to adapt to the specific role require-ments of 'parent of a handicapped child'.[28] However, observation of parents with handicapped children fails to lend much support to the view that, as a category, they occupy roles that are qualitatively different from those of other parents. The 'normal family', against which the family with a handicapped child is compared, is an abstrac-tion rather than social reality. Within a general framework, families face a wide variety of problems. Consequently, the role tensions faced by the family with a handicapped member are probably not so very different from the tensions created by many other circumstances which may affect families. Farber has referred to the existence of role organisational and tragic crises in families with a handicapped child.[29] Role organisational crises occur when the usual pattern of roles in the family is unable to cope with the additional demands made by a handi-capped child. Tragic crises, in contrast, are less a response to the practical problems of caring for a handicapped child but more a result of frustrated aims and aspirations. Farber suggests that role organisa-tional crises are more common among lower-class families, whereas tragic crises are more common among middle-class families. Whilst there are some differences between families from different social classes in the problems experienced in caring for a handicapped person, these should not be allowed to obscure the similarities. The pattern of domestic role organisation in middle-class families in our society only differs in minor respects to that in lower-class families. It is probable that families differ more in the way in which problems are presented to outsiders rather than in the precipitating factors. The basic problems of caring for a handicapped child revolve around practical issues of daily living and this should not be forgotten in a search for psychological and social deficiencies in the family. As far as these practical problems are concerned, middle-class families tend to be better equipped to cope with them because they are better off financially.

The effects on the family in its relations with the outside world can be usefully separated into short-term and long-term. The former concern day-to-day interaction between family members and others in the community, whilst the latter refer to the social mobility of parents and siblings.[30] Research studies have consistently reported limitations on extra-familial relationships. Holt found that 40 per cent of parents interviewed were unable to go out together, and other studies have reported, similarly, that families' social contacts and outside activities were limited.[31] However, the major deficiency in all of these studies is that no comparisons with 'normal' families were possible. Hewett concluded from her study, comparing 'normal' families with those with a cerebral palsied child, that there was no evidence to suggest that the presence of a handicapped child radically altered normal patterns of joint outings for the parents.[32] It seems likely that parents of handicapped children have similar patterns of social contacts to parents of any young child, although there are likely to be additional problems for the former in terms of how the child and the family are presented to outsiders.[33] It seems inadequate to think simply in terms of a limitation of social contacts. A study comparing mothers of normal children with mothers of mongol children found that both groups went out as much as they wanted to and reported that over 70 per cent of the latter welcomed the interest of strangers in their handicapped child.[34] Since the normal families in this study, and in Hewett's study, all had children below five years of age, it seems likely that social isolation and restriction of activities are experienced and expected by parents of young children in general, particularly by mothers. The differences between normal families and those with a handicapped child may, however, become apparent as the children grow older. The retarding influence of the handicapped child on the family cycle, and therefore the restrictions on parental activities, become more apparent as he or she grows older. Most parents expect their social lives to be curtailed whilst their children are young but they expect this to be a temporary situation, maybe ten or fifteen years at the most.

Studies of the long-term effect of the handicapped child on extra-familial relationships are concerned with the family's position in the social structure. A study of the social mobility of parents of severely mentally handicapped children in Chicago showed that the earlier in the marriage the child was born the more likely this was to have a depressing effect on social mobility.[35] Thus it was suggested that the handicapped child had an effect on the potential for upward social mobility, rather than causing downward mobility. However, there is insufficient evidence to conclude that the child influences social mobility. The fact that families of the severely handicapped are found to be evenly distributed among the social classes suggests that any effect on social mobility is slight. In a recent study, 6 out of 97 families reported that the father's career had been affected by the handicapped child, but the sample was biased towards the higher social classes and there was no means of checking the responses.[36] Whether or not social mobility is affected can only be established through careful longitudinal studies.

Practical Problems

What can broadly be termed the practical problems faced by families have often been neglected, although they have received more attention in recent years. Studies by Hewett, Bayley, Jaehnig and Carr have described in some detail the day-to-day practical problems that have to be faced and how these are dealt with.[37] The difficulties of feeding and changing nappies for a twelve year old, managing an aggressive child on public outings or doing the housework in the presence of a child who requires constant supervision are not very glamorous areas for the research worker, but the studies mentioned above have shown how important they are for families who have to cope with these problems every day of their lives. Hewett looked at the day-to-day problems of physical care, management, supervision, etc. of families with a cerebral palsied child and demonstrated their real meaning to the people most affected. She emphasised that, although the problems faced by these families were different and more severe than those of families with only normal children, the approach adopted by the parents in dealing with these problems was the same.[38] Problems of incontinence, feeding or temper trantrums were not treated differently because the child happened to be handicapped — the approach may have been modified but the rules were essentially the same. When Carr compared mongol children and normal children between the ages of 0 and 4 years, she found that, although the mothers of the mongol children did experience more problems in some areas, the only serious practical problem reported was feeding.[39] All children under five years of age present considerable management problems. They have to be trained to walk, talk, feed themselves, go to the toilet, wash, dress, etc., and this training is all carried out in the home. Thus the findings of the two studies mentioned above probably reflect the age ranges of the children in the studies. It might be expected that, as the children grow older and the discrepancy between the handicapped and the normal children becomes greater, the mothers of the former will identify a bigger range of practical problems. In the early years the objective problems presented by the handicapped child can be interpreted in a framework of normal expectations concerning the problems of caring for young children, but this becomes progressively more difficult as the child grows older but fails to develop. Changing nappies for a twelve year old is physically, psychologically and socially far removed from changing nappies for a two year old, or even a four year old. If the problems of caring for a severely handicapped adolescent are far removed from those of caring for a young child, the daily burden experienced by the family caring for a similarly handicapped adult is in a qualitatively different category.[40] Not only are the problems far more severe, but the capacity of the family unit and the individuals within it to deal with these problems is lessened. Siblings of the handicapped person have grown up and left home and the parents are getting older. It is important that the practical problems of day-to-day living experienced by families should be described, since it is with these ordinary daily tasks that services for the mentally handicapped can provide the most direct and effective support.

Material

There are two ways in which the handicapped person may have an effect on the family's material standard of living. On the one hand, the earning capacity of either or both parents may be reduced, and on the other hand, meeting the needs of the handicapped person may cause the family additional expenditure. The possible depressing effect on social mobility and therefore on the earning capacity of the father was mentioned above, but the effects on the mother's employment prospects are likely to affect a larger number of families. Jaehnig reported that, although a similar proportion of mothers of handicapped children as those in a control group was working, none of the former was working full time compared with 11 per cent of the latter.[41] In addition 14 per cent of the mothers of handicapped children said that the child had affected their work. Whether or not the mother goes out to work can make an important difference to the family's standard of living, but apart from restrictions on their income many families with a handicapped member find that they have many additional expenses; incontinence aids, special clothing, replacement of worn and damaged furnishings, special equipment, modifications to the house and extra transport costs.

It is very difficult to establish exactly how much the handicapped child affects the family's standard of living; consequently research findings in this area tend to be somewhat contradictory. Tizard and Grad's study, conducted in the late 1950s, found that families with a handicapped child at home were significantly worse off than those in which the child had been admitted to an institution.[42] However, the differences seemed to be due to the fact that the latter group of families were one member short, and therefore better off financially. A follow up study of the same families with a handicapped member at home five years later found that their position had deteriorated; 60 per cent had a limited income or found it difficult to manage.[43] One of the difficulties about making any judgement on the basis of these figures is that there is no opportunity to make any comparison with families who did not have a handicapped child. Jaehnig's more recent study did attempt to compare the families studied with a control group, and concluded that the former were worse off financially.[44] They were also shown to be worse off than a group of families whose handicapped child had been admitted to an institution, but the fact that the families were drawn from different geographic areas makes it difficult to draw any conclusions. Finally, in Carr's study the housing conditions of families with mongol children were compared with those of families who had only normal children, with the conclusion that the former were slightly better off, although the differences were not statistically significant.[45]

Thus the evidence concerning the impact of the handicapped member on the family's standard of living is somewhat contradictory. It is clear, however, that the handicapped member does present the family with financial problems which would not otherwise be incurred. Potential earnings of the parents are often reduced, many families find they have to spend more on clothing, consumer durables such as washing machines become necessities rather than luxuries, damaged furniture, etc. has to be replaced, and getting around either requires a car or the use of taxis. This additional burden has been recognised since 1973 with the introduction of the Constant Attendance Allowance, but it is difficult from the statistics available to calculate what proportion of parents with a mentally handicapped family member is receiving the

allowance. Another development in recent years which has helped ease
the financial burden for many families is the £3 million fund for
congenitally handicapped children administered through the Joseph
Rowntree Memorial Trust. However, whilst welcoming the provision of
this money, one must have reservations about the fact that it is a
limited sum and that not all families with handicapped children are
eligible for awards.

What should be clear from this brief review of findings concerning
the effects of the handicapped person on the family is the difficulty of
drawing any firm conclusions on the basis of so much conflicting
evidence. The family with a handicapped member faces certain special
problems and usually attempts to deal with those problems in the same
ways as would any other family, but the variety of these problems is
almost as large as the number of families. Whilst generalisations about
the needs of families with a mentally handicapped member must be
aimed at in order to plan benefits and services, it is not possible to use
generalisations to predict the problems of any particular family or the
effects that any one handicapped person might have. Support for
families should be related to the way in which they experience their
own problems and their own particular needs, and can only be effective
if based on an understanding of what family care means in practice.

What Does Family Care Mean

The White Paper, *Better Services for the Mentally Handicapped*,
emphasised the continuing importance of the family as the basic unit of
care for the severely mentally handicapped, but it did not have much to
say about what family care actually means. It is often too easy when
talking about community care to forget that what this means is feeding,
changing nappies, going to the shops, cleaning, cooking, etc. The
activities of daily living, the ordinary child care and domestic work, are
what constitute the nuts and bolts of community care, and they are
carried out by individual family members. The implication of the term
'family care' is that all the family members participate equally, or at
least participate to some degree, but implicit in the use of the term
'family' are a set of values and assumptions which make this unlikely.
The roles of individual family members are socially prescribed in the
family with a mentally handicapped member as in any other family, and
therefore the burden of care cannot be assumed to be carried by the
family as a whole. The distribution of this burden has received little
systematic attention, either from research workers or professionals
working with families, but an understanding of the actual mechanics of

family care is essential for the development of a satisfactory system of community care.

A number of authors have made reference to the role of the father in the care of the handicapped child. Schaffer suggested that fathers of handicapped children tend to be more involved with children than would be expected in most families in our society, but studies that have looked directly at the participation of fathers have not, in general, confirmed this view.[46] Hewett found no difference in the reported level of participation of fathers between families with a cerebral palsied child and those with only normal children, half of the fathers being described as 'highly participant' in both groups.[47] Similarly, Carr found little difference between the fathers of mongol children and other fathers.[48] Bayley's study of families with a mentally handicapped adult reported that 40 per cent of fathers contributed 'much help'.[49] Thus, on the evidence available, it would seem that about a half of fathers of handicapped children have 'high' levels of participation in child care and domestic work, and that this is approximately the same as for fathers of non-handicapped children. Hewett asked mothers whether the father engaged in a number of child-related activities, 'often', 'sometimes' or 'never' and, on the basis of this information, classified fathers as having 'high', 'medium' or 'low' levels of participation. It is not clear how these terms were defined and, in any case, such classifications are likely to be dependent on mothers' expectations of fathers as well as on the amount of work actually done. In addition, only child-related activities were considered, thus excluding all aspects of housework which constitute a major part of the domestic routine. The assessments used by Bayley were even less explicit and seemed to be based on his own impressions. Apart from the examples that he quotes, one cannot obtain much idea as to the frequency with which fathers actually performed tasks in the home. It may well be true that fathers of handicapped children provide as much support for their wives as do fathers of non-handicapped children, but to describe this as 'considerable' without reference to the overall amount of work which has to be done is misleading.

The role of siblings in the domestic routine of the family has received even less attention than that of fathers. Of the major studies of families with a handicapped member, only Bayley mentions the importance of siblings of the handicapped person in the domestic routine.[50] In one of the families he studied, two sisters had virtually assumed the position of mother, but in the remaining cases siblings played only a small part in the care of the handicapped person.

However, Bayley makes no reference to the extent to which they participated in other aspects of the daily routine in the home. Clearly siblings of the handicapped family member constitute an important potential source of support, although this may be limited to childhood and adolescence. More information on the importance of siblings as actual sources of support is necessary.

Support from the Community

The distinction between care *in* the community and care *by* the communuty is an important one.[51] It is evident that the care of most severely mentally handicapped people takes place in the community; what is not so clear is whether this is also care by the community. When considering community support for families, it is useful to make a distinction between formal support, i.e. that provided by statutory and voluntary services, and informal support, i.e. that provided by relatives, friends and neighbours. The former has received much more attention from policy-makers and researchers, but surely the latter is no less important, particularly since what emerges from the studies that have looked at the provision of formal services for families with a mentally handicapped member is that these services have a very small impact on the majority of families.

Formal Support

Tizard, in a review of services and the evaluation of services, comments that although education and to a lesser extent residential services have received a fair amount of attention, much less work has been done on the evaluation of other services.[52] There is a tendency, particularly among policy-makers, to emphasise institutional provisions and to equate evaluation with assessments of how close provisions are to certain prescribed and often arbitrary norms. There is a notable lack of attention to services provided directly to families, partly because the achievements of such services are less obvious and there are no convenient yardsticks which provide for evaluation. Perhaps the most common failure in the evaluation of services has been that the recipients, in this case the families, are not asked how they feel about the support (or lack of support) that they have received. A number of recent studies have, however, gone a long way towards rectifying this problem by presenting parents' detailed experiences of their dealings with the services.[53]

Bayley, referring to the experiences of families with a mentally handicapped adult, comments that the training centres were much appreciated by families because they provided structural help which was directly relevant to the daily routine. Nevertheless, only one third of the adults were actually attending training centres.[54] The families gave the impression that help with the small details of the daily routine would really have made a difference, but even when such help was provided, which was not very often, its effect was lessened by the fact that it was usually irregular and unreliable. Jaehnig also commented on the importance to families of the handicapped children's attendance at school, because this constituted direct support with the daily routine. However, like Bayley, he noted the marked lack of services, other than education, which had any impact on day-to-day problems in the home, and emphasised that where services were available to families they were oriented to crisis intervention rather than to the provision of long-term support. He concluded that 'Professional workers expressed little interest in the situation as long as the child was at home and the parents were not complaining'.[55] The impression of services given by Bayley and Jaehnig is representative of most studies which have attempted to evaluate services from the family's perspectives rather than measuring them against arbitrary levels of provision laid down by policy-makers. An analysis of the needs of families who approached the Family Fund for help revealed a great scarcity of contact with official services and reported that many families were not receiving the services they needed and were entitled to expect.[56]

However, it would be wrong to suggest that there have been no improvements in services during the past two decades. Education for the severely mentally handicapped child has improved, both in terms of the number of places available and the quality of provision.[57] The introduction of the Constant Attendance Allowance, already referred to, has benefited many families, and more short-term residential accommodation is available. It is unfortunate that the improvements that have taken place have failed to bridge the gulf between what is needed and what is available.

Although the development of adequate community services is hindered by a general shortage of resources, there are also other factors which inhibit their development. Where resources are available they are not always used to provide the sorts of services that families want and need. The discussion earlier in this chapter on the effects the handicapped person has on the family stressed the dangers of making assumptions about the family and denying their own legitimate perceptions of their circumstances and their needs. A study conducted in the United States attributed the overall direction of development in services to the emphasis among research workers and professionals on the psychodynamics and social psychology of the impact of the handicapped person on the family.[58] Professionals and research workers have tended to focus on their own definitions of the needs of families rather than being guided by the families' felt needs, with the result that the gap between what parents expect and want and what they actually get has widened. The same is true in this country, although perhaps to a lesser degree. The content and organisation of services is often based on professional evaluations of what is best, modified by bureaucratic considerations, what the professionals are able to offer and the power struggles that go on between different professional groups. Not only do services often fail to respond to the expressed needs of their clients, but also there is often little agreement between the professions themselves on what services should be provided. Jaehnig comments: 'Social policy for the handicapped is not the implementation of a commonly agreed upon platform of society's professional judges but the outcome of conflicting viewpoints of interested groups.'[59] Wing stressed the fact that each of the families she studied met the situation in a different way. Only through a close understanding of the individual circumstances and the needs felt by families themselves can an adequate service structure be developed.[60]

So far this discussion of formal support for families has made no mention of the various voluntary agencies, which often make a considerable contribution in terms of both advice and practical help.[61] Younghusband *et al.* commented on the outstanding contribution of voluntary organisations, and concluded that: 'Their role in the future may change but it is unlikely to diminish.'[62] Two of the main reasons for the success of voluntary groups are, first, that they tend to be more closely in touch with the needs of families than the statutory service , and secondly, that they attempt to fill some of the gaps left by the statutory services. The fact that families themselves are often involved in the running of these organisations and that professional interests tend to be less influential also makes them more responsive to the day-to-day problems of families. However, whilst they have an important role to play they cannot be a substitute for statutory basic services, which modern society should provide for families as of right rather than as a privilege.

Informal Support

In elaborating the theory and practice of community care, policy-makers, professionals and research workers alike have tended to emphasise the network of statutory and voluntary services. Although the 1959 Mental Health Act marked a significant turn towards care in the community based on the family, it failed to recognise the existing structures of support that families might already have. The emphasis was upon community care based on a network of services which would support the family. The role of the community in the form of relatives, friends and neighbours was sadly neglected, but the people who formulated government policy were not the only ones to make this mistake. Tizard and Grad's study, published in 1961, made no mention of the support which families received through informal networks, although Leeson, writing at about the same time, did stress the importance of informal networks.[63] She pointed out the dangers of rehousing policies which failed to take any account of the informal supportive networks some families were able to rely on in their present communities.

The 1971 White Paper was an improvement on existing policy statements, in that the importance to families of informal networks was recognised in the general principles: 'Understanding and help from friends and neighbours and from the community at large are needed to help the family to maintain a normal social life and to give the handicapped member as nearly normal a life as his handicaps permit.'[64] Unfortunately, this is the last of fifteen general principles in the White Paper, and no further mention is made of informal community support. More attention has, however, been devoted to this type of support by research workers in recent years. Michael Bayley describes three different levels of care by the community and states that 'the small scale level of the intimate, face to face relationships of the social networks of kin, friends and neighbours can be seen to be the basis on which care at the large scale level depends'.[65] In his interviews with families he gathered information on how this level of care by the community operated in practice; he reported that 70 per cent of families received 'considerable' support from neighbours.[66] Jaehnig also stressed the importance of social networks, but reported lower levels of support than Bayley; 60 per cent of families were receiving 'frequent' support from relatives but only 41 per cent were receiving some help from neighbours.[67] Similarly, Carr reported that over half of the mothers of mongol children she interviewed had a 'good deal' of support from relatives and friends.[68] Another study, in Northern Ireland, of families whose child suffered from cystic fibrosis, reported that 89 per cent of mothers were given practical help of one sort or another by their family or friends and about a third of mothers relied on relatives or friends to help with their domestic routine.[69] The overall impression generated by these studies is that the majority of families with handicapped members are able to rely to a considerable extent on relatives, friends and neighbours for support with the daily routine. However, when reading these findings, certain doubts spring to mind. Were the neighbourhoods studied typical of the social environment most families find themselves in? Exactly what tasks did people help with and how often? How did the support provided compare with the total needs of the families? It is likely that patterns of support were different in the communities dealt with in the three studies although it is difficult to say whether or not they were representative of different types of urban communities found in Britain today. But it is the methods of assessment of community support which lead one to express most concern over the validity of the findings. In all the studies assessments were subjective and relative to other families in the particular study. Either the researcher's or the respondents' subjective assessments were used. Terms such as; 'occasional', 'frequent', 'much', 'considerable' and 'a good deal' were not defined in ways which make it possible to repeat the assessments or to make comparisons; and distinctions between what people 'could do', 'would do' and 'did do' were not clear. The reader of these research reports can make comparisons between families in the individual studies but he has no means of establishing the relationship between what support was provided and the overall burden which constituted the daily routine for the families studied.

In summary, the approach of policy-makers and research workers to the role of informal community support for the mentally handicapped and their families leaves a lot to be desired. The former have tended to see the development of services in complete isolation from the wider social milieux in which families care for their handicapped member, whilst the latter have countered this neglect with an almost naive enthusiasm for the idea of supportive communities. The reality for most families is by no means clear. What is clear is that informal support can be very important, but it is necessary to place this support in perspective by relating it to the overall burden experienced by family members.

Home Care or Institutional Care?

Although the majority of the severely mentally handicapped, particularly children, are cared for in their families, the White Paper estimated that there were over 66,000 such people in institutions and that a further 9,950 institutional places would be required.[70] The conditions many of these people experienced have been highlighted by Pauline

Morris and by the enquiries carried out at Ely and Farleigh Hospitals.[71]
Conditions in hospital and residential care for the mentally handicapped have improved in the last ten years although there is still a long
way to go. It is not my intention here to discuss in any detail the
problems of institutional care; my focus is on a consideration of the
factors which make it more or less likely that families will seek long-
term institutional care for a handicapped member. One of the prime
objectives of a policy of community care is to enable the family,
through the provision of supportive services, to continue caring for
their handicapped member for as long as they wish. In many cases the
decision to seek long-term residential or hospital care is precipitated by
situations which, had the family received appropriate support at an
earlier stage, might have been avoided. It is therefore important to look
at factors associated with families' decisions to seek long-term care in
order to establish what types of services would help them to care for
the handicapped person for as long as they wanted to. Much of the
early work on factors related to admission to long-term care was done
in the United States, but more recently attention has been devoted to
this question in the UK. It is convenient to separate factors related to
admission into three different categories; those concerning the handicapped individual, family factors and community factors.

The Handicapped Person

There is general agreement that the severity of the individual's physical
and mental handicap is the most important single element in the decision to seek institutional care. Tizard and Grad found that 62 per cent
of their institution sample of children had social ages of below three
years compared with 25 per cent of their home sample, which is consistent with most other British and American studies.[72] Apart from the
degree of handicap the other major factor concerning the handicapped
person is the presence of behaviour problems, particularly behaviour
problems which occur outside the home.[73] One study referred particularly to 'anti-social' and 'immoral' behaviour as major factors which
lead families to seek long-term care.[74] It may be that the emphasis on
the handicapped person's social behaviour outside the immediate family
is an aspect of the more general problem of visibility. Tallman has
argued that acceptance and adaptation of the family to the handicapped child is related to the visibility of the handicap.[75] Where the
child can very easily be recognised as mentally abnormal, either through
physical appearance or through social behaviour, it may be more
difficult for parents to manage encounters in public, particularly with

strangers.

Other characteristics related to admission are the age and sex of the handicapped person. Not surprisingly, most studies report an increasing rate of admission with age.[76] A recent survey indicated that, by the time children reach the ten to fourteen age group, most low grade children have been admitted to long-term care. At five years of age less than one-third of all severely mentally handicapped children are in institutional care, but by fifteen years of age this has risen to a half and by thirty-five to four-fifths.[77] Not only do the physical problems of caring for the severely mentally handicapped person in the family increase as the child grows older, but the ability of ageing parents to cope with the problems may decline, and siblings of the handicapped member, who may have provided support in the past, tend to leave home and have families of their own to care for. In addition to these factors, the behaviour of the handicapped person tends to deviate more and more from what is socially accepted. Strangers find it much more difficult to accept child-like behaviour from an adult, and what might have once been regarded as endearing in a young child often becomes embarrassing in an adult. Thus a whole range of factors conspire to bring pressure to bear on the family to seek long-term care as the handicapped child becomes a handicapped adult. Within this pattern there is also a greater likelihood that boys will be admitted rather than girls, and at an earlier age. Although the fact that boys tend to be larger than girls, and therefore physically more difficult to handle, must play a part in this, cultural factors are probably more important. A recent study suggested that there is a greater acceptance of deviance on the part of girls, and Olsen noted that sex differences in admissions are directly related to cultural expectations which provide a more protected atmosphere for females.[78] Since boys are expected to be more active and to achieve more than girls, the discrepancy between the handicapped boy and his normal peers is more noticeable. Whether gradual changes in sex role stereotyping of children will have any effect on this pattern remains to be seen.

The Family

A considerable amount of attention has been devoted to the relationship between the structure and conditions of the family and the decision to seek long-term care. The birth order of the handicapped child appears to have some bearing on whether or not institutional care is sought. A number of British and American studies have reported that first born children are most likely to be admitted and last born least likely.[79] One of the studies of mentally handicapped adults carried out in this country reported that 46 per cent of the adults left at home were last born children, compared with only 18 per cent who were first born.[80] Farber and others in the United States have suggested that parents are better able to cope with the handicapped child if there are already normal children in the family, and that the tendency to keep the child at home if he or she is the last born is a result of infantisation (i.e. creating a permanent baby) of the handicapped child.[81] In some families the birth of a handicapped child at the end of the child-rearing period provides a not entirely unwelcome opportunity for the parents to continue to care for a small child almost indefinitely. However, there are contradictory elements in the various studies relating family composition to the decision to seek long-term care. Hewett found more first born handicapped children at home than in hospital, which is somewhat surprising in the light of the findings of the studies reported above.[82] As far as family size is concerned, some studies report that larger families are more likely to seek institutional care and others that smaller families are more likely to do so, which suggests that the cultural context may be an important variable. The influence of family size may be completely different for a working-class family in Sheffield and a middle-class family in St Albans. Clearly the standard of living experienced by the family is likely to have some bearing on the decision. Two of the most recent studies in this country report poorer material conditions among families institutionalising their child than among those keeping him or her at home.[83]

Evidence concerning the parents of the handicapped person is also somewhat contradictory. Hewett reported that mothers who were over 30 years of age at the time the child was born were more likely to admit the child, but other studies have found that younger mothers are more likely to seek institutional care.[84] Bayley found that institutionalised children in his sample were more likely to have younger mothers whilst adults were more likely to have older mothers.[85] The explanation for this discrepancy may lie in changes in the roles of women and their social expectations, which will receive more discussion in later chapters. There does seem to be general agreement among the various studies that mothers whose health is poor are more likely to seek admission of their child to long-term care, and that marital breakdown is also likely to lead to long-term admission.[86] Similarly, it has been reported that parents whose child is admitted are more likely to have poor marital relationships, although these have not finally broken down.[87]

There are certain problems, however, in much of the information connecting family factors with the decision to seek long-term care since the wishes of the family may not be decisive. Professionals are, to a large extent, responsible for deciding who shall and who shall not be admitted to the long-stay institutions. Differences between families whose child is admitted and those whose child remains at home must partly result from the views that the professionals have about which families are 'capable' of caring for the handicapped person and which are not. This is particularly the case in relation to assessments of marital and family relationships. Given the emphasis in professional models on the pathological consequences for the family, referred to earlier in this chapter, it is hardly surprising that there is a tendency for professionals to identify problems among those families who seek institutional care for their handicapped member. What is surprising though is the fact that research workers have often failed to question professional evaluations. Thus one study based classifications of marital relationships on assessments made by social workers after admission had taken place,[88] and another found that a significantly higher proportion of mothers whose child was institutionalised reported marital disruption.[89] The former of these two studies relied on professional judgements and both were retrospective, therefore providing no means of establishing whether these evaluations reflected *post hoc* justifications of the decision to seek long-term care. Bayley, reporting more generally on family relationships, found that more of his institution group suffered problems according to social workers.[90] In the light of the over-emphasis in the literature on the family with a handicapped member on pathological consequences, it is hardly surprising that there is a tendency for professionals to identify problems in family relationships, particularly where institutional care is being sought.

In contrast to the stress laid on family relationships as a factor precipitating institutional care, relatively little attention has been paid to the importance of practical aspects of the organisation of care within the family. Those studies that have devoted some attention to these problems have suggested that they can be important elements in the equation leading to the decision to seek long-term care for the handicapped person. Hewett reported that fathers of children admitted to long-term care were significantly more likely to be described as non-participants in child care and housework than fathers of children not admitted.[91] Similarly, Jaehnig found that parents in his home sample were more likely than those in his hospital sample to adopt a joint pattern of conjugal roles rather than having carefully defined responsibilities for husband and wife, which usually meant that the husband played little or no part in child care and housework.[92] These studies suggest that the organisation of the domestic routine in families and the extent to which family members contribute might be an important factor in deciding whether, or at what age, long-term care should be sought for a handicapped family member. There is, however, a need to devote much more attention to these questions, thus shifting the focus from emotional and psychological factors to practical problems, which might be more amenable to solutions other than the drastic step of seeking long-term institutional care.

The Community

The relationship between the decision to seek long-term care for the handicapped family member and the amount of support obtained from outside the family has received some attention, particularly in recent years, but this has hardly been proportionate to its importance. Since the essence of current policy for the severely mentally handicapped is to encourage community care based upon the family and to create a supportive environment which will enable families to keep the handicapped person at home for as long as possible, knowledge of the relationship between levels of community support and admission to long-term care is vital. Saenger, in a study carried out in the United States, found that, when families in home and institution samples were matched on characteristics known to be related to admission, low grade cases remaining at home had received a significantly higher level of services than the institution sample. He concluded that the provision of more community services would reduce the demand for institutional care.[93] However, the relationship between the provision of better services and the decision to seek long-term care is somewhat more complex in practice. A study in this country considered the relationship between increased provision of training centre facilities and the demand for hospital care. The authors reported that demand for hospital care had declined over a period in which training facilities had improved, but they also noted that further improvements in the facilities did not produce a further decline in demand, and that there was no relationship nationally between improved training facilities and demand for hospital care.[94] More recent studies by Bayley and Jaehnig have looked at the relationship between the provision of a wide range of services and admission to hospital, but in neither study was the evidence very conclusive. Bayley commented that, although no hard conclusions could be drawn, 'where there was a lack of the sort of care and support which would enhance the life of the family, there was an association with admission to hospital'.[95] Jaehnig, however, found that the level of support received by all families was very low and that there was not a great difference between his home and hospital groups in the services received. In respect of short-term care, the hospital group had received more provision prior to admission than the home group were receiving at the time of the interviews. He attributed such differences to the tendency of the services to respond to crises rather than provide continuing support.[96]

If the relationship between the provision of community services and the decision to seek long-term care has received inadequate attention, that between the levelof informal community support and the decision to seek long-term care has been almost totally neglected. The studies by Bayley and Jaehnig are the only ones which seem to throw any light on this subject. Bayley, however, was unable to say much about the importance of informal support since the files from which his information was gathered made little mention of this aspect of family life. There was no information available for over half the families, but among the remainder many more families where the handicapped person was at home were receiving a fair amount of support than those from which the child had been admitted to hospital.[97] The fact that little mention was made of informal sources of support in the records is significant in itself, since it reflects the tendency of service providers to see the services as the major providers of support and to take little account of informal networks. Jaehnig reported that informal support, in common with support provided by the services, was very limited when compared with the total needs of the families. Nevertheless, he did find a marked difference between home and hospital groups. Only 12 per cent of the latter had three or more sources of support compared with 42 per cent of the home group.[98] One should, however, treat these findings with some caution. Methods of assessing community support were criticised earlier in this chapter and it will become apparent in later chapters that there is a very great difference between an occasional helping hand and regularly available support with the daily domestic routine. There is a great need for much more precise information concerning the relationship between formal and informal sources of support for families and how these affect the family's ability to continue caring for a handicapped member.

Conclusions

The past 30 years has seen the growth of a large body of literature on the subject of families caring for severely mentally handicapped people.

Parents, teachers, doctors, social workers, researchers, politicians and many others have contributed to the wide ranging debate, which has undoubtedly improved our understanding of the experiences and needs of the family caring for a handicapped person. Perhaps the most important message has been simply that the success of policies designed to care for the mentally handicapped in the community depends on the families who undertake the burden of care, although it is not always obvious that this has penetrated to those responsible for planning and developing services. Whilst the increased attention given to the problems of families is a welcome step forward, there has, however, been an over-emphasis on certain aspects of family care and a relative neglect of others. Many professionals (doctors, social workers, psychologists, etc.) and researchers have viewed the family with a handicapped member within the framework of a pathological model, resulting in an over-emphasis on the psychologically and emotionally damaging effects on family members and insufficient attention being paid to the practical problems of caring for a handicapped person. In contrast, a number of books and articles by both parents and research workers have, in recent years, attempted a different approach to the problems of such families. They have maintained that they are essentially the same as any other family, but that they face special problems with which they require practical help. They tend to adopt the view that practical help is usually necessary and that the provision of such help will often remove or alleviate psychological and emotional problems, although some families will continue to need help with these.

Whilst much more attention has been devoted to the needs of families there remains a lack of the detailed information on the mechanics of care in the family and the relations between the family and the rest of the community that is necessary to construct a picture of the reality of community care. There are a number of useful anecdotal descriptions written by parents and other descriptions of care in the community by research workers. Unfortunately, the latter have failed to provide a systematic analysis of how care in the family is organised and, although they have described levels of informal community support, have not related this support to the burden experienced by individual family members. Since the prime objective of pursuing a policy of community care is to enable families to continue caring for the handicapped person for as long as possible, it is necessary to obtain detailed information about how the burden of care is distributed, in what ways this is related to decisions to seek long-term care for the handicapped person and how those most involved in caring feel about their problems.

3 AIMS AND METHODS

Government policy since 1959, at least at the level of principle, has clearly asserted that community care is the most desirable form of care for the majority of severely mentally handicapped people. Although this has always been the predominant form of care, it has not always been accepted as a desirable alternative to residential or hospital provision. Many people hoped that once the principle of community care had been accepted this might lead to the development of more effective community services to support the handicapped individual and his or her family. Unfortunately, although there have been certain improvements in the past 20 years, the provision of community services has lagged a long way behind statements of principle. Although the inadequacy of the finance made available was a major factor in this lag, a further reason for the failure to develop effective services was an inadequate and sometimes non-existent appraisal of exactly what was meant by community care in day-to-day practice. Policy statements are based on certain, usually implicit, assumptions about the nature of the family and the community. The family is often referred to as though it is a total caring unit, no mention being made of the different roles played by individuals or how these might or might not be changing in modern society. The community (although attempts are rarely made to define the term) is expected to provide practical, emotional and social support for families. From the point of view of policy-makers with limited resources at their disposal, such assumptions are perhaps convenient; from the point of view of families with a handicapped member they are often far removed from reality.

Professionals in regular contact with families have often made the same mistake as policy-makers in devoting insufficient attention to the day-to-day mechanics of care in families and their sources of support. They have tended to concentrate on other less mundane aspects of the problem of care, and to see themselves as primarily serving the needs of the handicapped individual rather than the family as a whole. Research workers have, in general, devoted more attention to the practical problems of care in the family, the relevance of services to families' needs and the role of the community. However, even they have not always avoided making the same mistakes as the policy-makers. They have, for example, made little attempt to achieve an understanding of exactly what constitutes care in the family on a day-to-day level, and they have failed to treat the issue of who does what in the family as problematic. Attempts have been made to assess the contributions to community care of relatives, friends and neighbours, but since these assessments were not related to any estimate of the overall burden of care they are of limited value. How can we plan effective services without an adequate understanding of what care in the family really means, how much support is provided by the community and by the services, and how in turn this support is related to the burden of care experienced by the individuals in the families?

The family is taken for granted as the unit of care, but families consist of individuals, and the way in which the burden of care is distributed within the family is important. Thus the study described in this book was designed to look at day-to-day care of the handicapped person in the home in the context of the remainder of the family's domestic routine, and to relate this daily domestic routine within the family to outside sources of support. Where family and external resources were inadequate, an additional objective was to assess the need for additional support with the daily routines. Finally, the study was designed to examine decisions about seeking long-term residential or hospital care. The current policy of encouraging care in the family for as long as possible rests on the untested assumption that support provided to the family will improve ability to cope, and therefore lessen or delay the likelihood of the family seeking long-term care for the handicapped member. It was hoped to explore whether this assumption is justified for most families.

It was pointed out in the previous chapter that families with a severely mentally handicapped member are essentially the same as any other family. They are not somehow independent of the wider social fabric; social changes and pressures affect them as much as they affect any other family. Theoretical and empirical studies of the family and its social environment in modern British and American society have thrown some light on the problems of caring for the severely mentally handicapped in the community. Therefore, before describing the approach adopted in this study, it is useful to consider the relevance of research that has been conducted on normal families. Of particular relevance is research which has looked at patterns of role relationships within the nuclear family, whether these are changing and the relationships, in modern society, between the nuclear family, kin, friends and neighbours. In addition, it is important to review the meaning and utility of two concepts which are central to the implementation of current policies for the mentally handicapped but which, nevertheless, are usually ill defined; the concepts of community and need.

Role Relationships in the Family

Before proceeding to a discussion of roles in the nuclear family it is essential to clarify what sociologists mean by the term role and to elaborate on the relevance of a study of role relationships in the family to the problems of caring for a mentally handicapped family member. The social world of the individual can be viewed as a network of inter-locking social systems, e.g. family, work, social club, political party. Each system consists of a group of statuses which are the positions which individuals occupy within the system. Thus any individual can occupy many different statuses at the same time in different social systems e.g. father, employee, councillor, etc. Each status carries with it a set of behaviours which are expected of the person occupying that particular position and these constitute a role. Roles exist independently of the particular actor and, although there may be scope for individual interpretation, behaviour is prescribed within certain broad constraints. Whilst there is scope for variation, certain behaviour, such as attending meetings and acting on behalf of constituents, is expected of a councillor if he is to continue to occupy the status. The behaviour prescribed for any particular status may vary between different social groups at the same time and over time within the same social groups (e.g. the behaviour expected of a working-class father in relation to child care may be very different from that expected of a middle-class father. Similarly the role of all fathers in child care today is not the same as it was in the nineteenth century.) Families with a mentally handicapped member are faced with a modified set of role relationships for two reasons. First, the handicapped person is unable to fulfil normal role obligations, and second, the problems experienced by the family exceed normal expectations.

As the normal child grows up, his or her role inside and outside the family changes as new patterns of behaviour are learned and depen-dency on adults declines. The mentally handicapped child is unable to keep pace with these changes and usually remains very dependent on care and supervision from adults. He or she is thus granted an alterna-tive status, and the aspects of the roles of other family members which relate to the handicapped person are modified accordingly. How the roles of mother, father, brother, sister, etc. are interpreted in ordinary families and those with a mentally handicapped child can be very important in terms of who carries the burdens of child care and housework which constitute the day-to-day reality of community care.

Clearly, the principal focus of attention must be on the definition of marital roles and from the point of view of this study, on the domestic division of labour. This is an area of investigation which has been badly neglected by sociologists, although it is perhaps not surprising that a profession dominated by men should concern itself with issues deemed important by men. The domestic division of labour has not usually been one of these. To the extent that sociologists and others have concerned themselves with the family and what goes on inside the family, they have largely accepted the sexual division of labour between husband and wife as given. Child care and housework have traditionally been regarded as maternal role obligations and sociologists have, in general, seen little reason to study the effects of the predominant patterns of role organisation in the family, or to question these patterns. Legal, social, psychological and economic factors do much to create a situation in which the role of wife or mother is tied to the role of unpaid domestic worker. In contrast, the man as breadwinner, figure of authority and envoy to the outside world, is not expected to participate in the domestic routine. This differentiation between the roles of female and male is central to the structure of the family in modern society. The clearly defined role of the woman in the family in a traditional coal mining community was described in *Coal is Our Life*, written in 1956. The wife must:

> . . . in a very consciously accepted division of labour . . . keep in good order the household provided for by the money handed to her each Friday by her husband. While he is at work she should complete her day's work – washing, ironing, cleaning or whatever it may be.[1]

Are there reasons to suppose that the position of women in the family and the domestic division of labour is changing? The study quoted above was conducted more than 20 years ago in a type of community that was already declining and which has since become the exception rather than the rule. Working-class communities, in which men worked long hours in physically demanding and sometimes dangerous occupations whilst their wives worked even longer hours raising large families, have given way to more mixed urban communities composed of smaller, more affluent families in which most men work shorter hours in less physically demanding occupations, whilst their wives often have paid employment of their own. The position of women outside the family has certainly undergone some important changes in the past 30 years. In 1950 only a quarter of women were in employment compared with about half today, of whom two-thirds are married. Changes in attitudes towards women at work have been reflected in legislation to achieve equal pay and equal opportunities, although there remains a gulf between good intentions and economic realities. In a more general way, the growth of the women's liberation movement has challenged existing attitudes and practices. As far as the family itself is concerned, the introduction of the contraceptive pill in the early 1960s gave women a degree of control over child bearing that they had never before possessed. Such changes took place alongside a rising standard of living and increased ownership of domestic appliances. All these developments have, individually and collectively, been interpreted as signs of women's increasing emancipation from the home, and therefore from domestic drudgery. Whether the changes are merely symbolic or whether they reflect a real change in the status of women is, however, open to question.

The first point to make in assessing the impact of wider social and economic changes on familial roles and on the domestic division of labour is that there is no necessary connection between the two. Legislation to ensure that women are not discriminated against in their occupations is, for example, no guarantee that they will be freed from discrimination in the home. The participation of women in the labour force in certain geographic areas, in certain industries and at certain times has been higher than it is today, but there is no evidence to suggest that a high level of participation in the labour force has had much bearing on the definition of familial roles. Legislation cannot ensure equality of opportunity within the family. Modern domestic technology might be thought to have transformed the position of the woman in the home by reducing the overall amount of domestic labour, but this assumes that housework is a finite task. However, any housewife can tell you that the housework is never done, no matter how many domestic appliances she has or how many convenience foods are available. In order to obtain an accurate assessment of the domestic division of labour there is no substitute for a direct analysis of the organisation of child care and housework in the family. Only in this way is it possible to assess whether or not changes in familial roles have take taken place.

Most modern sociological studies of marriage have stressed the relative equality of husband and wife today as compared with the nineteenth or earlier twentieth centures.[2] Young and Wilmott recently reported that, when wives worked outside the home: 'In the interests of symmetry it was only fair, as husbands and wives saw it, for the men to do more so that their wives could do less.'[3] It is suggested by such studies that there is not only a tendency for the husbands to do more in the home but also for marital roles to become less precisely defined and differentiated between husband and wife. In Elizabeth Bott's terms, there is an increasing tendency towards joint marital roles and away from segregated roles.[4] The trend is supposed to be most apparent among middle-class families but it is said to have become increasingly common among working-class families also. However, a number of studies have questioned the way in which the concepts are used and the validity of conclusions based on limited empirical studies.[5] To classify marital role relations on a single dimension (e.g. joint — segregated) seems limiting, to say the least, and there is no good reason to suppose, as seems to be suggested, that joint decision-making or joint financial arrangements imply joint participation in domestic tasks. Oakley's recent study of housework sharply questions assumptions about increasing symmetry and jointness in marital relationships in so far as the domestic routine is concerned. She found that, when she asked what husbands actually did as opposed to what they should do or would do, the reported level of participation was very low, 60 per cent being recorded as having a low level of participation in housework.[6] The questions she used were carefully constructed to establish exactly which domestic tasks husbands actually performed and how often. In contrast, Young and Wilmott based their conclusions about increasing symmetry in domestic marital roles on vague questions and little reference to the overall burden of domestic work. Their conclusion, that role relations in most marriages are tending towards symmetry, seems to be based on the fact that 85 per cent of fathers helped with at least one household task at least once a week![7] What is meant by symmetry seems to be a slightly increased level of help given by men in child care and housework, but remaining within the bounds of a sharply defined sexual division of labour. The best available evidence indicates that in the vast majority of families, women still carry the burdens of child care and housework with only limited support from their husbands.

So far no reference has been made to the contributions children make in many families to the domestic routine. The main reason for this relative neglect is that virtually all studies of the organisation of domestic labour tend to ignore the contribution of children. They are assumed to be dependent and therefore only to contribute to the equation in a negative capacity, but the contribution of older children to the care of their younger siblings and to housework can be as great, and often greater, than that of their fathers. The larger nineteenth-century family relied heavily on the participation of the children, mainly girls, in child care and housework. Although the modern nuclear family is smaller, and older children are therefore less likely to have younger siblings, their participation in housework may be very important. If Oakley's conclusions about the relatively low level of participation of most fathers are correct, it is likely that some teenage children contribute at least as much as many fathers.

What are the implications of all this for the family with a severely mentally handicapped member, and does the presence of such a person result in a redefinition of familial roles to cope with an exceptional situation? It was pointed out earlier that studies of families with a handicapped member have not, in the main, regarded the organisation of domestic labour as an important focus of study, and where they have devoted some attention to it have unquestioningly accepted traditional assumptions about the nature of the family and the roles of women. Such an acceptance is hardly surprising in the light of the fact that a traditional sexual division of labour in the home is fundamental to the operation of the welfare state. The health care system in particular is based on the availability of care for the sick person in the family. Only in exceptional circumstances does the health care system take over the physical care of the sick person, and even then it is usually only for short periods. The family is responsible for the hour-by-hour care that precedes admission to hospital and/or follows discharge. The person who is usually expected to make herself available to administer the care necessary is the wife/mother. In the case of chronic conditions, such as mental handicap, the care that has to be provided does not have the same time limits as are expected in the care of the acutely ill person. Nevertheless, mothers are still expected to be available to provide this care. The policy of encouraging care in the community for the chronically sick person is based on assumptions about the ability of families to meet the demands placed upon them which, in practice, usually means the willingness of mothers to carry the burden of care. There is no evidence to indicate that families in this position undertake a major redefinition of familial roles; it is more likely that in most such families the mother carries an even heavier burden than usual. A system of care which thus exploits a particular section of the community is not only morally unacceptable, but may also find itself increasingly undermined if changes in the social role of women outside the family produce changes in expectations which begin to make themselves felt in the home.

The Relatively Isolated Nuclear Family

The nuclear family does not exist in social isolation. The vast majority of British families live in urban communities and are potentially able to call on the support of relatives, friends and neighbours in addition to statutory and voluntary services. The relationship between the modern nuclear family and its social environment has been the subject of considerable debate among sociologists. In particular, this debate has dealt with the importance of kinship networks. The structural functional school argues that the nuclear family predominates in modern industrial society, principally because its characteristics bear the best fit with the demands of a modern economic system. It is argued that economic, political and social functions, once allocated to the extended family, have been taken over by the differentiated institutions of modern society. Thus socialisation of children is increasingly undertaken by the educational system, and the care of the sick is undertaken by the health care system. It is not my intention here to discuss alternative theories of the family but the functionalist position, crudely outlined above, has produced the now widely held view that the modern nuclear family is isolated from the contacts with wider kin which are characteristic of families in pre-industrial societies. If this is so, the implications for any family caring for a severely mentally handicapped member, or any other chronically sick person, are considerable, since kinship networks have traditionally been utilised to mobilse support for the care of the highly dependent.

The specific point of departure for most of the discussion on the question of the relevance of kinship networks to the modern nuclear family was an essay by Parsons on the kinship system of the United States.[8] In this essay he described the 'isolated conjugal family' as the normal household unit in American society. He suggested that the social and geographic mobility demanded by the modern economic system results in a weakening in the strength and salience of ties of birth and kinship. However, the critics of the functionalist view have produced a considerable body of evidence which shows the continuing importance of kin networks as a source of support to the nuclear family in industrial societies. Laslett challenged the basic assumption of the functionalists, that the nuclear family is more prevalent in modern industrial societies than it was in pre-industrial societies. He showed that the proportion of families in Tudor England who had resident in-laws was smaller than that among families in Bethnal Green in the 1950s.[9] Similarly, Anderson showed that members of the extended family outside the domestic unit in nineteenth-century England become *more* rather than less important as sources of support in dealing with critical life situations such as ill health, death, unemployment, etc.[10]

In the present century, demographic change, affluence and the advent of the welfare state have reduced the frequency and changed the nature of the life crises that affect most people. A higher standard of living and better medical care have reduced the death rate at all ages, unemployment and retirement benefits have cushioned the effects of losing one's job and insurance may soften the blow caused by events such as loss of possessions, fire or accident. Consequently, whether or not links are maintained with kin has become a matter of choice rather than necessity. Most families face fewer crises today and their resources for meeting these problems are much better, but their needs for long-term support have not declined and may even have increased with the rise in the numbers of chronically sick and old people. The findings of Young and Wilmott show clear evidence that, at least in Bethnal Green in the 1950s, a three generational family system existed and that this was not merely based on sentiment, but on a high degree of mutual aid and support.[11] Similarly, Townsend found that 58 per cent of the old people he studied were members of three generation extended families, although many lived separately from their children.[12] The apparent contradictions between these findings and the arguments advanced above may be resolved on closer examination. Although the demographic, economic and social changes referred to have been taking place throughout this century, the biggest changes have taken place since the Second World War. For the majority of working-class families in pre-war Britain, ill health and unemployment were never very far away and, although the state provided a basic level of support, additional support from family and friends was a necessity rather than a luxury. The families studied by Young and Wilmott and by Townsend in the 1950s belonged to working-class communities with traditions of mutual support going back to the depression of the 1930s and earlier. Increasing affluence, high employment, the development of health and welfare provisions, large-scale re-housing, increased geographical mobility, etc. have radically altered the circumstances of most families in the past 20 years. There is a need to re-assess the importance of kinship networks in the light of such changes.

Much of the evidence concerning the kinship networks of nuclear families in modern industrial societies is based on American research. Lytwak and Sussman and Birchenall have argued that kinship links remain important for the majority of families.[13] They argued that it is not the isolated nuclear family which is characteristic of modern societies but the modified extended family. They emphasised the considerable autonomy of family units but, at the same time, their partial dependence on other family units within a network. This network seems to exist in both middle-class and working-class families. A study by Bell, in this country, of middle-class families during the early years of marriage found that they maintained contact and received support from relatives even when they were geographically mobile.[14] However, Bell noted that less support was available with regard to child rearing than might be the case in families less geographically separated. The trend seems to be towards more flexible relations with kin and, whilst mutual support is still important, the nature of this support has changed as the circumstances and needs of families have changed. But for the family with a severely mentally handicapped member the nature of support is crucial. Support is required on a day-to-day basis with the mundane chores which constitute the domestic routine. There is no reason to suppose that changes in the level and nature of support from kinship networks do not affect the family with a handicapped person as much as any other family. If this is so then it means that these families are becoming less and less likely to receive the sort of continuous support which they need.

Only kin have been mentioned so far in this discussion, and it is true that most of the contributions to the debate on the social relations of the nuclear family have concentrated on the importance of kinship groupings. Litwak and Szelenyi, however, have included kinship groupings, neighbourhoods and friendships in a general discussion of primary groups in urban industrial society.[15] Although such primary groups tend to operate in different ways, they suggest that not only do they survive, but they may also perform some functions more efficiently than bureaucratic agencies. Similarly, Bott has argued that families in modern urban societies are not isolated, but possess social networks of variable densities which can be utilised in meeting crisis situations.[16] If it is true that social groups other than kin are significant for the nuclear family in modern society, it is important to include them in any assessment of supportive social relations. Informal support can be seen to be provided by social networks of varying sizes and densities alongside that available to the family from bureaucratic agencies. It is clear that certain agencies, such as the health service and the educational system, fulfil some specialised functions which would not commonly be expected of the social network, but there may be a considerable degree of overlap in the provision of direct supportive services to the family in the home. Obvious examples of this are: the sort of advice and support provided by social workers; the practical support with the domestic routine provided by a home help; assistance in finding suitable housing; and help with transport. In addition, support provided outside the household, such as residential or hospital care, may serve some of the same functions as support that might otherwise have been provided by relatives or friends in the family's own household. The evidence that is available with respect to families with a handicapped member suggests that, where overlap between social network and service support does exist and a choice is available, the former is often judged to be preferable to the latter.[17] This implies, however, that the nuclear family, the social network, and the services are overlapping systems rather than interlocking parts of the same system, the system of 'community care'. Is there any sense in which a community can be said to exist which is more than the sum of its individual parts?

The Concept of Community

The term community care has already been referred to many times in this book but no attempt has so far been made to analyse the meaning of the word 'community'. Since the objective of the study described in this book was to examine the day-to-day practice of community care, it is important to devote some attention to the conceptual meaning of the term community. Plant, in an essay on community and ideology, stresses the difficulty of arriving at any agreed definition; 'Community is so much a part of the stock in trade of social and political argument that it is unlikely that some non-ambiguous and non-contested definition of the notion can be given.'[18] The term is not without some descriptive meaning, but its evaluative component is considerable. The supposed demise of the community and its replacement by a rational 'association' has been a major concern of social scientists since the nineteenth century. Tonnies illustrated the evaluative component when he pointed out that, whilst it is possible to talk of bad society (*Gesellschaft*), to talk of bad community (*Gemeinschaft*) violates the meaning of the word.[19] His book, *Community and Association*, published in 1887, was an indictment of the baneful effects of many of the features of modern life. He contrasted *Gemeinschaft*, in which human relationships are intimate, face-to-face, involving the whole person, with *Gesellschaft*, in which relationships are discrete, segregated and circumscribed by a sense of specific obligations. Thus, community is something to be positively valued, but what is its descriptive meaning? It has been linked by various authors to the locality, identity of functional interests, a sense of belonging, shared ideas and values and a way of life

opposed to the bureaucracy of modern mass society.[20] However,
although there is overlap between various definitions of the term, none
of these characteristics is an essential component of all definitions.
Locality is a commonly accepted but not universal feature; Webber's
definition of interest community, for example, does not require
spatial proximity.[21] Thus, scientists, trade unionists, students,
religious groups, etc. might all be considered to be communities in some
sense of the word. Minar and Greer sum up what can be said in general
of the term: 'Community is both empirically descriptive of a social
structure and normatively toned. It refers both to the unit of society as
it is and to the aspects of that unit that are valued if they exist and
desired in their absence.'[22]

If the concept of community is itself highly problematic then what
do we mean when we talk of community care? The report of the Committee on Social Workers in the Mental Health Services (the Mackintosh
Report) used the term community care more than 25 years ago, and
since then it has been applied to many different groups of people
requiring care.[23] But this report and subsequent White Papers and
government reports failed to make any attempt to define the term. It
was not until 1968 that an official document made some attempt to
define community. The authors of the Seebohm Report, whilst being
aware of the difficulties of defining the concept, noted that 'the notion
of community implies the existence of a network of reciprocal social
relationships, which, among other things, ensure mutual aid and give
those that experience it a sense of well being'.[24] If it is care in this sort
of community that is advocated by policy-makers few would argue with
its desirability, but many would question whether it does, or even can,
exist for the majority of people in modern urban society. In practice,
the use of the term community in social policy in this country seems to
have meant nothing more than the majority of the population who do
not live in residential institutions. Its use seems to have had little to do
with a positive, value-laden approval with which it is often endowed,
except in so far as policy-makers have relied on these connotations as
a means of winning approval for the policies. It is possible that the use
of the term was intended to foster the development of a form of care
which would have these favourable connotations, but the failure to
specify in detail and plan the development of the sorts of services
necessary has produced a practical reality which is very different from
the theory. Community care has come to mean care outside of an
institution, or sometimes care in special sorts of rather small institutions which are located in areas of residential housing. Thus the term

community seems to have little value either as a conceptual tool or as a device for describing a specific type of service. For the purposes of the study described in this book, therefore, the concept of community has no meaning other than the sum of its parts; the family, the social network, the services.

The Concept of Need

The definition of need presents a central problem for the health and social services. The objectives of these services can only be defined in terms of the needs of the groups and individuals they serve, and ultimately the only criteria for a satisfactory evaluation of services is the extent to which they meet the needs of their clients. Needs are constantly referred to in official documents, books, articles, speeches, etc., but few attempts to define the usage of the term are made. Whose needs are being defined and on what basis are they being assessed? The first of these questions may not at first sight seem very important, since the answer might be expected to be the patient or client's needs. However, whilst it is quite clear whose needs the surgeon operating on the victim of a road accident might consider foremost, it is not so clear whose needs the social worker dealing with a family with a severely mentally handicapped child should consider. The tendency of the professions dealing with the mentally handicapped to identify the handicapped person as the only, or at least the principal, client has shifted more recently to an emphasis on the family as a whole. Whilst it is clear that a conception of the family as a unit has to be maintained, such a formulation is often insufficiently explicit. Although the family as a group can be said to have certain requirements or needs, there are many areas in which it is necessary to consider the needs of individual family members. The preceding discussion of the modern family stressed the fact that a sexual division of labour continues to exist in the vast majority of homes and that the day-to-day domestic routine remains a maternal responsibility. It is therefore necessary to view needs associated with this routine as predominantly the needs of one individual, i.e. the mother. Although other family members also have needs which may at times conflict with the needs of the mother, only through an understanding of needs of individual family members is it possible to consider the family as a whole.

Providing an answer to the second part of the question (i.e. on what basis should needs be assessed?) is more difficult. Forder, in a useful discussion of the problem, identifies six different methods of assessing needs: ideal norms, minimum standards, comparative need, felt need,

need defined according to specific techniques and national need.[25] When needs are defined according to an ideal norm, an optimum standard is set which is not necessarily obtainable but against which measurements can be made. A classic example is the WHO definition of health as 'a state of complete physical, mental and social wellbeing and not merely the absence of infirmity'. The meaning of a minimum standard definition is fairly obvious; needs are assessed according to a basic standard which it is considered all people should achieve. Minimum standards laid down for housing are an example of needs defined in this way, although the standard changes over time. Comparative definitions are an extension of minimum standards. Instead of defining a minimum level through supposedly objective criteria, the standard is set by comparisons with the average, e.g. the provision of day places for the mentally handicapped should not be below the national average. Felt needs make use of the individual's subjective feeling of discrepancy between what is and what ought to be, but of course they rely on the individual being aware of this discrepancy. It should, however, be remembered that felt needs are not always translated into expressed need, even if individuals are asked, which often they are not. One of the commonest approaches to the definition of needs is to abandon goals and to define needs according to the specific techniques available. Thus we might talk of the need for kidney machines, psycho-therapy or social case work. Finally, national need can be regarded as the sum of the needs of all the individuals comprising the nation. It is at this level that the needs of one group are weighed against the needs of another, the need to provide better health care may be weighed against the need to provide full employment.

Each of the methods of defining needs outlined above has its advantages and its disadvantages, and it would be wrong to suggest that one should always be used in preference to others. Different approaches are appropriate to different situations and often in the same situation, but it is important that the method being used is clearly specified, thus allowing for the fact that there will be alternative approaches to the particular problem. Whilst it is desirable, for example, to bear in mind the definition of health based on an ideal norm mentioned above, this may not be very helpful in providing practical solutions to particular health problems. If we consider the situation of people suffering from rheumatism, it might be helpful to define their needs in various ways: through comparisons with standards of care provided for other groups; through asking them what they feel they require; through a consideration of the relative merits of contributing more resources to this group

as opposed to others; or through establishing the numbers who would
benefit from the specific treatments available. Each of these methods
will produce a different assessment of the needs of this group, but they
are all valid approaches to the problem. All too often needs are
presented as absolutes, when in fact they are relative to the particular
method of assessment used.

With regard to the health and social services in general, and the care
of the severely handicapped in particular, there has been an over-
emphasis on certain approaches and insufficient attention paid to
others. Although ideal standards and comparative definitions have
played their role at the level of general statements of policy, the actual
development of services reflects much more the use of definitions based
on the specific techniques available. Ensuring that the mentally handicapped have the same rights as other members of society must be a
long-term objective for services. In the meantime needs must be defined
taking into account many other considerations. What this has meant in
practice, very often, is that needs for particular services have been
assessed such as hospitals, training facilities, social case work and
behaviour modification.

At times it has appeared that it is principally the needs of professional groups that are being served, rather than the needs of the clients.
As new professions have become prominent a greater need for their
services has been discovered, thus providing employment for the professionals. However, there are other ways of defining needs which have
received little attention from policy-makers or professionals, but which
can provide practical approaches to short-term problems. In particular,
the needs felt by clients themselves have often been ignored or have
received scant attention. It is true, as mentioned above, that clients will
not always be fully aware of the possibilities or of how their situation
compares with that of other people or with certain ideal standards, but
it is arrogant to insist that their perception of the situation is irrelevant
and that only a qualified professional worker is capable of identifying
the clients' needs. One of the few studies of social work practice from
the clients' perspective commented:

To offer clients, such as those studied, psychological help – without
satisfying, and preferably at the start, their material needs – in our
view utterly fails to come to grips with their problems . . . It is
absurd to expect that the urgency of their needs could be met by a
non-material approach, whether this be a matter of offering insight,
providing friendship, or the opportunity to unburden themselves to a

sympathetic listener. Plainly put these individuals were desperately in need of money (or its equivalent) and to offer them something else is to offer a suit of clothes to a drowning man.[26]

For the present study it was considered important to look at the clients', in this case the mothers', perceptions of particular aspects of thier situation, partly to redress the balance and partly because it was assumed that these would be most relevant to the decision to seek long-term institutional care for the handicapped family member. More specifically, mothers' perceived needs for additional support with the various aspects of the daily domestic routine constituted the focus of attention. This is not to imply that the mothers, and other members of the family, do not have many other needs, which they may or may not experience as such, but this research focuses on the burden carried by one individual in the family and her feelings about it, since it is hypothesised that these are highly relevant to her ability to cope with the situation.

The Handicapped Person

So far I have referred, in the main, to families with a severely handicapped member, making no distinction between children and adults. There are good reasons for studying the process of community care in the family with respect to severely mentally handicapped people of all ages. However, in this study, it was decided to include only families with a severely mentally handicapped child (i.e. under 16 years of age) for four main reasons. First, as mentioned earlier, there are far more mentally handicapped children than adults living with their families. Most severely mentally handicapped children live with their families whilst for adults, particularly those over 30 years of age, this becomes less and less common. Secondly, the problems experienced by families with a handicapped child are closer to those of other families, since all children are expected to be dependent to some degree. Thirdly, although the family cycle is already distorted by the prolonged babyhood of one of its members, it has not yet reached the point where, if it were not for the handicapped child, all the children would have become fully independent. In other words, the family with a severely mentally handicapped chld is not too far removed from the situation in which most families find themselves. Finally, one might expect that support from the social network would be more readily available for families with children, since the family is still in a position which is in accord with the expectations of outsiders. Relatives, friends and neighbours might be expected to make a greater contribution to the family with a

severely mentally handicapped child simply because families with
young children are expected to require support from outside.

Summary of Objectives

At the beginning of this chapter the objectives of the study were outlined. In the light of the subsequent discussion and before moving to a
description of the study itself and the methods used, it is possible to
summarise the principle objectives of the study. It was hypothesised
that:

1. Community care predominantly means care within the family
with varying degrees of support from relatives, friends and
neighbours and from formal services.
2. The organisation of child care and other aspects of the domestic
routine within the nuclear family reflects traditional definitions of
familial roles, which are based on a sexual division of labour, and,
therefore, family care predominantly means care by the mother.
3. Many mothers feel the need for additional support with child care
and housework.
4. Ability and willingness to cope with the severely mentally handicapped child, indicated by whether or not long-term care is sought is
related to: (a) the receipt of support with the domestic routine from
other members of the nuclear family; (b) the receipt of formal and
informal support with the domestic routine from outside the nuclear
family; (c) the perceived needs of mothers for additional support
with the domestic routine.

Put more succinctly, the objective of the study was to describe the
process of community care and the relationship between levels of
support and felt needs and the decision to seek long-term institutional
care. Inevitably such a study must highlight inadequacies in existing
levels of support, both formal (services) and informal (relatives, friends,
neighbours). Thus a fundamental objective of the study was to establish
how services for the mentally handicapped and their families, and more
particularly for the mothers of mentally handicapped children, could be
improved in order to begin to provide the sort of support that would
really justify the term community care.

Methods

The findings of this study, described in later chapters, are based upon
structured interviews with 120 mothers of severely mentally handi-

capped children. Half of the mothers had a severely mentally handicapped child who was awaiting admission to long-term hospital or
residential care and the other half were not, as far as was known,
seeking long-term care for their handicapped child. In all cases the child
was living at home at the time the interview was conducted. The
families whose child was awaiting admission were spread over the whole
of the greater Manchester conurbation and the others all lived in
Salford. The interviews covered a wide range of topics which have been
classified under the following headings: the handicapped child, the
mothers, other family members, participation and support in the daily
domestic routine, the services, and felt needs for additional support.

The Samples

For reasons of time and resources available the samples were restricted
to 75 in each group giving a total of 150 possible respondents. The
sample of families in which the handicapped child was not awaiting
admission to long-term residential care, hereafter referred to as the
home group, was drawn from Salford County Borough. The Salford
Psychiatric Case Register provided the best sampling frame of severely
mentally handicapped children available locally. The sampling frame
was 116 children on the register who were not already in long-term care
or known to be awaiting admission and the sample was drawn using
random numbers. The mental handicap section of the case register has
been in operation for a number of years, and links with local services
are very good, most cases being identified at an early age. Salford, at
the time of the survey, had a population of about 110,000. It is a
densely populated industrial city which forms part of the greater
Manchester conurbation. In terms of the social class composition of the
population, the lower social classes are over-represented, since many of
the people in non-manual occupations who work within the city
commute to work from the suburban areas outside the borough.

The selection of a sample of families whose child was awaiting
admission to long-term residential or hospital care presented more
problems. Since the focus of the study was on the daily domestic
routines of families caring for a severely mentally handicapped child, it
was important that the handicapped child was living at home at the
time the interview took place, but it was equally important that the
family should have taken the decision to seek long-term institutional
care. The obvious source from which to draw such a sample was the
waiting lists for admission to a mental handicap hospital, but there was
some doubt regarding the significance which could be attached to the

presence of the child's name on the waiting list. Therefore, a small pilot study of families whose child was on a waiting list was conducted. In all cases the parents were aware that the child's name was on the waiting list and were actively seeking a long-term hospital or residential care place. Consequently it was decided to draw the sample of families whose child was awaiting admission, hereafter referred to as the admissions group, from the waiting lists of the three main mental handicap hospitals serving the Greater Manchester area. The medical directors of all three hospitals agreed to supply names and addresses of children on their waiting lists on condition that the introductory letter to the mothers, although drafted by the researcher, was sent to parents by the hospitals, and that the mothers were given the option of declining the invitation to participate by returning a reply-paid postcard to the hospital. The waiting lists of the three hospitals produced a total of 60 children whose names had been placed on the lists within the preceding five years.

Since the admissions group drawn from the hospitals waiting lists was 15 short of the target of 75, it was decided to obtain a further sample of families from those awaiting admission to local authority residential care. Manchester Social Services Department was approached with this in mind but had no waiting list of a formal nature. However it was suggested that individual social workers would be able to supply the names of children who were awaiting long-term care or who were likely to be admitted to long-term care in the very near future. Accordingly, a letter was sent to all social workers in Manchester asking them to provide names and addresses of severely mentally handicapped children in this category. The response to this letter produced a total of 18 names, three of whom were excluded because the child was found to be over 16 years of age.

The children whose names were referred by social workers constituted a slightly different group from those whose names were drawn from hospital waiting lists. First, their names were not formally present on any waiting list and secondly, they were more likely to be admitted to local authority residential care than to hospital, but in most respects they were similar to the group drawn from the hospital waiting lists.

As far as the representativeness of the samples is concerned, the home group and the admissions group are best dealt with separately. The sample of home group children from Salford can be assumed to be representative of children on the mental handicap section of the Salford Psychiatric Case Register. The Register is well established and has built up good links with the medical, social and educational services. The fact that it has a very good coverage may mean that the home group in the present study was more representative of the local population of severely mentally handicapped children than were the samples that have been used in some other studies. The rather higher numbers of children identified as severely mentally handicapped in Salford compared to other areas is probably due to more comprehensive coverage and to the identification of children at an earlier age than is possible where there is no standard procedure for collecting information.

The representativeness of the admissions group is a much more difficult problem to assess. It was apparent from the variable sizes of the waiting lists maintained by different hospitals that waiting lists are somewhat arbitrary and are very dependent on such factors as the admissions policy of the hospital, liaison between hospital and social services, the provision of alternative forms of accommodation and the nature of the hospital's catchment area. Similarly the sample referred by social workers was probably influenced by arbitrary factors. There is, therefore, no basis on which to judge whether or not these groups were representative of all the children in greater Manchester who were likely to be admitted to long-term care in the next few years. Nevertheless, this was a group of children who were very likely to be admitted to long-term care in the near future, and it seems reasonable to make comparisons between this group and the home group which is representative of all severely mentally handicapped children living at home.

Initial contact was made with mothers through an introductory letter which explained the purpose of the research and asked them if they would be prepared for an interviewer to call. The overall response rate of 80 per cent was satisfactory although not quite as high as had been expected. In particular, the response rate for the home group (83 per cent) was disappointing. More than half of the non-responses in this group were due to refusals or failure to keep appointments. Previous interviewing experience with families of the mentally handicapped had led to an expectation of a very small number of refusals. The higher number of refusals in this study was probably due to the fact that many of the mothers in the home group had been interviewed in connection with research at least once in the preceding two years. However, the response rate achieved was still satisfactory and the evidence available gave no grounds for supposing that the families of the non-respondents were different from those actually interviewed. The response rate among the admissions group was 77 per cent. The lower rate for this group was in the main not due to refusals but to families having moved away from the area or failure to make contact.

Since the names of these children had been on hospital waiting lists for up to five years it was to be expected that some would have moved away, although their names had not been deleted from the lists.

The Questionnaire

The questionnaire, which was developed from a pilot study, was designed to gather information concerning the handicapped child, the parents, the families, informal support (relatives, friends, neighbours), formal support (service provisions), and the felt needs of mothers for additional practical support. Although the questionnaire as a whole was highly structured and pre-coded to facilitate analysis, a proportion of the questions was left open-ended in order to allow mothers to respond more freely. In addition, space was left for the interviewers to record fuller responses, even where the response categories were pre-coded. In most cases it took between 1½ and 2 hours to complete the interview schedule. In relation to most social research interviews this might appear to be an inordinately long period of time, but most mothers were only too willing to set aside the necessary time to talk about their handi-capped child, and in many cases the interviews had to be terminated because the interviewers had other appointments.

It would be tedious to describe the questionnaire at length, but the way in which certain topics were dealt with requires some discussion. All questions were designhned specifically for the requirements of this particular study, excepting those relating to the child's behaviour, skills and handicaps which were derived from a schedule developed by Dr Lorna Wing at the MRC Social Psychiatry Unit.[27] In its original version, this schedule was very comprehensive and had been tested on other populations, but was very detailed and took over an hour to administer. It was therefore considerably reduced for the present study, items being selected to provide assessments of the child's main handicaps and behaviour problems and his or her abilities. However, comparing children in terms of individual aspects of behaviour, such as mobility, speech development, play, ability to wash and dress, etc. does not enable one to establish a picture of overall levels of development. An assessment of intelligence was not considered appropriate, since IQ does not necessarily reflect social competence which has far more relevance to the family situation than intelligence. Social competence refers to the child's ability to wash, dress, feed himself, etc., to partici-pate in ordinary domestic routines and to play independently, etc. A test of these sorts of abilities was required in order to establish the degree of independence in relation to the tasks of child care and housework, the performance of which constituted the main focus of the study. There are a number of possible approaches to measuring social competence, each with their advantages and disadvantages.[28] It was decided to use the Vineland Social Maturity Scale and items were selected from the MRC schedule to facilitate the completion of this. The principal advantages of the Vineland Scale are that it covers a wide range of behaviours and provides an overall assessment of the child's level of social development which is easily understood. The scale is standardised for normal children and therefore provides an indication of the extent to which a handicapped child deviates from normal expectations. However, it should be borne in mind that any scale which reduces a child's level of development to a single figure is necessarily crude.

The importance of a careful and detailed analysis of the domestic routine has already been pointed out earlier in this chapter. A major section of the questionnaire dealt with this domestic routine in three sections; physical child care, child minding and housework. Pilot interviews with mothers and fathers had shown that a clear distinction was made between participation in a task and support with it. It was clear that there was a qualitative distinction between taking sole or shared responsibility for a task (participation) and providing help for the individual who took responsibility for it (support). Thus, in the questionnaire, mothers were asked who usually performed each task and then whether anyone else ever helped; the former were described as participants and the latter as supporters. Up to three individuals could be recorded as usually performing the task and up to four could be recorded as helpers. Thus a mother might say that she and her husband usually shared the washing up whereas she usually did the cooking and her husband only helped occasionally. In the first example mother and father would be described as participants, whilst in the second the mother would be a participant and father a supporter. The distinction worked very well in practice, mothers clearly made the distinction themselves between participants and supporters. Although further distinctions could have been made, particularly in the category of helpers, these would have required either very detailed questioning or asking mothers to keep a diary over a period of time, neither of which was practicable.

The other major problem area in terms of the design of the questionnaire was the method of measuring felt needs. For each of the 15 tasks which constituted the domestic routine, the mother's assessment of whether she needed additional support was required. It was found that when mothers were asked whether they *needed* additional support, very few replied that they did. By definition they did not need additional support, since in practice they were coping on a day-to-day basis without it, but many said they would have liked to have this additional support. Since most of them accepted that these tasks were maternal role obligations, to admit to needing more help would have been an admission of failure to meet obligations, and thus to have threatened their status as mothers. However, to admit that they wanted or would have liked more help involved no such threat. Thus they were not asked whether they *needed* additional support but whether they *would have liked* additional support. In the context of this study, therefore, an admission of wanting additional support was taken to imply felt need. In addition, a further distinction was made between those who felt that this additional help would have been very important and those who felt it was an optional extra. Accordingly, if the mother observed that she would like more help, she was then asked how important she felt it would be to have this extra help. In practice, mothers did not want help with all tasks, and those that they did want more help with they rated differently with respect to the importance attached to having this additional support.

To summarise, the study was designed to construct a picture of the day-to-day reality of community care for families with a severely mentally handicapped child. The emphasis was upon the experiences of the one individual in the family who carries the heaviest burden; the mother. Community care rests heavily on the willingness of mothers to undertake the domestic tasks which are what care is all about. The extent to which they are supported by other members of the family, by people outside the family and by the services, may make a great difference to their ability and willingness to cope with the problems. It is to be hoped that the descriptions contained in the following chapters of the problems that the mothers experienced will be given careful consideration by those responsible for the planning and delivery of services.

4 THE CHILDREN AND THEIR FAMILIES

The study was mainly concerned with the day-to-day domestic routines of the families and, more specifically, with the mothers and their experiences of caring for their handicapped children. However, the children so dominated the lives of many families that a detailed description of them is essential to understand the families' predicaments. In addition to this, of course, the extent of the child's handicap constituted one of the most important factors in the decision to seek long-term residential or hospital care. In this chapter the children in the home and admissions group are described and compared in terms of their sex, age, handicaps, skills and behaviour problems. In order to enable the reader to obtain a better understanding of living with a handicapped child, the bare descriptions are supplemented by the mothers' own accounts of their children's behaviour, which describe the problems in graphic detail. The remainder of the chapter is devoted to a description of the families and their circumstances, which were another important element in the decision to seek long-term care. The ages of the parents, the age, sex and number of other siblings, the family's standard of living and the adequacy of their accommodation all had a bearing on whether or not they felt able to cope with their handicapped child. In considering other family members, however, particular attention is focused on the mothers, since it is they who shoulder the major part of the burden of care. The effects of carrying this burden on their work and social lives, their health, their feelings and their expectations are crucially important for the future of the handicapped child and therefore whether or not the children are admitted to long-term care.

The Handicapped Children

Sex and Age

Studies of handicapped children in institutional care are consistent in reporting that boys are more likely than girls to be admitted.[1] In this study, where the sample for the admissions group was drawn from waiting lists, there was no marked preponderance of boys. There was a slightly higher proportion of boys than girls in both home and admissions groups but the differences between the groups were negligible.

There were, however, considerable differences between the groups in the ages of the children, which ranged between 2½ years and 16 years. Table 4.1 clearly shows the preponderance of older children in the admissions group, where only 19 per cent were under 8 years of age, compared with 42 per cent of those in the home group. At the other end of the spectrum 48 per cent of the admissions group children were over 10 years of age compared with 34 per cent of the home group.

Table 4.1: Age of Child

| | Age | | | | | |
	0-4 years	5-7 years	8-10 years	11-13 years	14-16 years	Total (100%)
Home	11 (18%)	15 (24%)	15 (24%)	14 (23%)	7 (11%)	62
Admissions	2 (3%)	9 (16%)	19 (33%)	19 (33%)	9 (16%)	58
Total	13 (11%)	24 (20%)	34 (28%)	33 (28%)	16 (13%)	120

In the home group the 0-4 and 14-16 age groups were under-represented. In the lower age group this may have been related to deficiencies in the diagnostic and assessment systems which resulted in some cases not being identified until after the age of five, but, since these systems were relatively well developed in Salford, the age distribution of the children may also reflect real changes in prevalence. The most recent evidence from the Salford Mental Handicap Register shows that the incidence of severe mental handicap rose during the mid-1960s and has since fallen.[2] The larger number of children in the 5-13 year age range in the present sample would be consistent with this pattern. In the admissions group the very small proportion of children who were between 0 and 4 years of age is probably due to a lower demand for residential care places from parents of younger children and an unwillingness on the part of the services to regard requests for institutional care of young children as legitimate. The number of children awaiting residential care reaches a peak between 8 and 13 years of age, declining thereafter as places are found. One might have expected that there would be a corresponding recruitment to waiting lists from children in the home group, but this was not the case. It is possible that waiting lists are utilised for children in the middle age range in order to legitimate the parental request for long-term care without actually providing a residential place. When parents seek a place for a child of 9 or 10 years of age the authorities may feel that, although the domestic situation is difficult, the child can be managed at home for a few more years. In the case of older children the home situation is more likely to have reached a point where it is impossible for the family to cope.

This chapter continues with a discussion of the relationship between the children's level of development and the decision to seek long-term care. However, the different age distribution in the two groups rendered straight comparisons difficult, since both the objective level of development and the family's subjective experience of problems vary with the age of the child. Severely handicapped children differ from normal children, not in that they are dependent, but in the degree to which they are dependent. The discrepancy between normal expectations and the handicapped child's actual performance increases as he or she grows older, and the objective management problems increase as he or she gets bigger. Thus a doubly incontinent four year old is not directly comparable with a doubly incontinent fifteen year old. For these reasons 'age matching' of the two samples was performed which made them directly comparable but reduced their size. Of the 62 children in the home group 46 were matched with individuals in the admissions group according to age. Thus 28 children were excluded from the subsequent analyses of handicaps and behaviour, leaving a total of 92, 46 in each of the two groups.

Health

Although, in general, children in the admissions groups were more likely to suffer poor physical health or impairments, such as loss of sight or hearing, than children in the home group, the differences were smaller than might have been expected. In terms of general physical health, 13 per cent of those awaiting admission were described as suffering poor health compared with 7 per cent of home group children, but a larger proportion of those in the home group were described as having only average health. Apart from the child's general health, mothers were asked whether he or she suffered from epileptic fits, and if so how serious these were. Whether or not they were classified as serious depended on the extent to which mothers felt that the fits presented a problem and disturbed normal domestic routines. Nine children in the admissions group were described as having epileptic fits of this nature compared with seven in the home group. Finally, two aspects of physical disability, eyesight and hearing, were felt to merit special attention, since problems in these areas can constitute a major compli-cating factor in relation to the child's other disabilities. Slightly more children in the home group suffered some visual problems but all of the four children who were blind or almost blind were among those awaiting admission to long-term care. The combination of severe mental handicap and blindness can be formidable. Gillian was 13 years old, fully mobile, but incontinent and almost blind. Her mother described some of her problems:

> It's the constant watching of her and the cleaning up of her. You have to be up and down stairs all the time to see that she has not gone into someone else's bed and wet that. She always has to be watched. She will sometimes walk into walls and doors. She goes up and down stairs but there is a constant danger that she might fall.

Hearing difficulties on the other hand did not appear to be related to whether or not the family was seeking long-term care. Of the three children who suffered moderate or severe loss of hearing, two were in the home group and one in the admissions group. In summary, it appears that there is no consistent relationship between aspects of the child's physical health, except perhaps blindness, and the decision to seek long-term care. Whether or not ill health, epileptic fits or problems with hearing constituted a major problem depended very much on the particular circumstances that the family experienced.

Disabilities

Information was obtained on a wide range of behaviour in order to obtain an overall assessment of the children's social maturity, which will be discussed later. Eight aspects of behaviour which are fundamental to daily living have been selected in Table 4.2. These provide an indication of the extent to which the children were capable of caring for themselves and playing a part in the normal domestic routine. In all eight aspects of development shown in the table, the children in the home group were more advanced than those in the admissions group.

Most of us expect our children to be able to get around without assistance from a very early age and we quickly take this for granted, but all of the 17 children in the admissions group in this study who were completely immobile were over 5 years old. Their inability to move around presented enormous problems of physical management. In one family the child could only be moved when both parents were present to lift him, and in another a downstairs room had been converted into a bedroom because it was physically impossible to get a 14-year-old girl up and down stairs. For some of these families the problems of physically moving a handicapped child constituted a major

Table 4.2: Disabilities

	Home N = 46 (100%)	Admissions N = 46 (100%)	Total N = 92 (100%)
Mobility			
Not mobile (unable to crawl)	1 (2%)	17 (37%)	18 (20%)
Mobile but unable to walk without support	15 (33%)	10 (22%)	25 (27%)
Walks without support	30 (65%)	19 (41%)	49 (53%)
Feeding			
Has to be fed or can only use fingers	4 (9%)	23 (50%)	27 (29%)
Uses implements but needs help	19 (41%)	10 (22%)	29 (32%)
No help necessary except with difficult food	23 (50%)	13 (28%)	36 (39%)
Washing			
Needs washing or can only wash hands	23 (50%)	29 (63%)	52 (57%)
Washes and dries hands and/or face	10 (22%)	9 (20%)	19 (21%)
Baths self with or without help	13 (28%)	8 (17%)	21 (23%)
Dressing			
Child has to be dressed	22 (48%)	30 (65%)	52 (57%)
Dresses with help	14 (29%)	12 (16%)	26 (28%)
Requires no assistance or only minimal assistance	10 (22%)	4 (9%)	14 (15%)
Continence (day)			
Frequently incontinent	12 (16%)	27 (59%)	39 (42%)
Usually reliable if taken	11 (24%)	7 (15%)	18 (20%)
Goes to toilet of own accord	23 (50%)	12 (26%)	35 (38%)
Comprehension of speech			
Little or no understanding	8 (17%)	26 (57%)	34 (37%)
Follows simple instructions	22 (48%)	10 (22%)	32 (35%)
Follows more complex instructions	12 (26%)	8 (17%)	20 (22%)
Able to understand information on topics outside experience	4 (9%)	2 (4%)	6 (7%)
Usual method of communication			
Does not communicate or gets what he wants	4 (9%)	22 (48%)	26 (28%)
Communicates through gestures or attempts words	22 (48%)	17 (37%)	39 (42%)
Makes requests in words	20 (44%)	7 (15%)	27 (29%)
Level of speech development			
Does not say any words	16 (35%)	30 (65%)	46 (50%)
Single words only	5 (11%)	5 (11%)	10 (11%)
Short phrases	13 (28%)	7 (15%)	20 (22%)
Talks in sentences	12 (16%)	4 (9%)	13 (15%)

reason for seeking long-term care, but alternative solutions to such problems were rarely suggested by the services. Most mothers had not even received advice about the best methods of lifting and carrying a child. Faced with a problem which can only become worse as the child grows heavier it was hardly surprising that most of these mothers saw long-term care as the only solution.

Large proportions of severely mentally handicapped children require at least some help in basic activities such as feeding, washing and dressing, but there is an enormous gulf between a child who has to be spoon-fed a liquid diet at every meal and the child who occasionally requires difficult foods to be prepared for him. Children in the former category were far more common in the admissions group, whilst children in the home group, although they required assistance, were not usually totally dependent. Differences between the groups were greatest in the area of feeding, where half of the admissions group were unable to use knives, forks and spoons compared with only 9 per cent of the home group. These children included some who could only manage a liquid diet using a special feeding cup. Sometimes feeding was further complicated by the child's refusal to eat certain foods or even to eat at all. Andrew was awaiting admission to long-term care, and feeding constituted a major problem for his mother:

> The last twelve months have been particularly difficult because Andrew refuses to eat or drink anything. He has had bouts of this before which lasted a few days but he was strong enough to get over them. If I force the food in he won't swallow. He got thinner and thinner and dehydrated very quickly until we had to send him to hospital where they feed him with tubes.

Differences between groups in respect of washing and dressing were smaller since these activities require a generally higher level of competence and greater motivation. Nevertheless, notably more of the home group children were independent in these areas.

One of the most difficult problems faced by mothers of severely handicapped children is that of incontinence. Although the majority of incontinent children were only incontinent of urine, a considerable minority were also incontinent of faeces. The practical and social problems of coping with incontinence were largely dependent upon the age of the child. Mothers of younger children tended not to identify it as a major problem, but for the families of older children life inside and outside the home often revolved around the problems of changing nappies, washing, getting rid of smells and finding toilets. Apart from the practical difficulties which increase as the child grows older, incontinence becomes less and less socially acceptable with age. Incontinence in an older child was frequently a major factor in the family's decision to seek long-term care. Of admissions group children, 59 per cent were frequently incontinent compared with only 26 per cent of home group children. Most mothers found it extremely difficult to obtain practical advice or support which might have removed, or at least eased, the problem. Even when practical assistance, such as the provision of disposable nappies, was available, it was often so difficult to obtain that many mothers did not bother. One mother decided to buy her own disposable nappies rather than obtain them through the health visiting service, since this involved a once weekly visit to a health centre and a wait of up to one hour only to find, sometimes, that the correct type of disposable nappy was not in stock.

The remaining three items in Table 4.2. deal with various aspects of the child's ability to communicate. The ability to understand and to be understood is a necessary precondition for the development of many other skills and for the development of relationships. A high proportion of admissions group children were severely deficient in all three aspects of communication dealt with in the table. Of these, 57 per cent had little or no understanding of speech, 65 per cent were unable to say any words and 49 per cent seemed to make no attempt to communicate through either speech or gesture. In contrast, only 9 per cent of children in the home group made no attempt to communicate. In some cases problems of communication overshadowed the difficulties of physical care. John's mother identified one major problem, although John was also incapable of dressing or washing himself:

His not understanding us and us not understanding him is the worst thing. You don't know what he wants from us or what he is trying to tell us. If he could communicate he could play with the other children, but they just make fun of him.

Social Responsiveness and Independence

The skills considered in the previous section concerned the child's functional capacity for independence; i.e. the extent to which he or she was capable of performing basic self care tasks and communicating with other people. However, functional independence is neither sufficient nor necessary to enable the child to develop rewarding relationships with other people and to engage in independent activities. Mothers were

asked how their child responded to affection and social communication
and whether he or she made spontaneous approaches to other people.
The ability to give and respond to affection is very important for the
development of satisfactory relationships. Many mothers found caring
for their handicapped children a very rewarding experience, but this
was so only when the children responded to their parents and other
people in a socially acceptable way. Even children with little or no
speech were in some cases able to give and respond to affection and to
communicate through other means. Home group children were more
likely than those in the admissions group both to respond to physical
and social approaches and to attempt to communicate their feelings
spontaneously. Only 4 per cent of home group children never showed
affection spontaneously compared with 28 per cent of admissions
group children, and although there were 16 children in the home group
who had no speech, only 5 of these made no attempt to communicate
spontaneously. In contrast 21 of the 30 similarly impaired children in
the admissions group made no attempts at spontaneous communication.

Not only were children in the home group more socially responsive
but they were also better able to amuse themselves than those in the
admissions group. Eighty per cent of them could be relied upon to
initiate some form of activity, even though this was often of a
repetitive nature. This meant that they could be left alone without
stimulation or close supervision for periods of time. In contrast, half of
the children in the admissions group never initiated any activities
themselves and three-quarters could not be left without close supervision. One of the most important preconditions for some degree of
independence is a basic understanding of everyday dangers but 76 per
cent of children awaiting admission had no such understanding. They
had no comprehension of the danger involved in touching a hot stove,
playing with sharp knives or falling from a height.

Social Maturity

So far in this review of the handicaps and skills of the children, selected
aspects of behaviour have been treated separately, but this does not
enable the reader to form an overall impression of the level of development and how this was related to the development of normal children.
The Vineland Social Maturity Scale was used to obtain an overall index
of each child's social maturity.[3] Scale scores were based on the level of
achievement in a wide range of behaviours, ranging from the ability to
sit unsupported to reading and writing. From the point of view of a
consideration of the problems presented by the handicapped child in

the family, such an assessment is more meaningful than an assessment of intellectual achievement, since it measures the child's actual performance in day-to-day activities in the home. Only 6 per cent of the handicapped children in the survey achieved social ages of more than five years but, within this general pattern, there were considerable differences between the two groups. Whereas only 7 per cent of children in the home group had a social age of below one year, 44 per cent of those in the admissions group were in this category. These children were unable to use a spoon for eating, required constant close supervision, were unable to drink from a cup unaided, and could not be relied upon to discriminate edible from inedible substances. At the other end of the spectrum, two-thirds of the children who had social ages of over three years were in the home group and, of the 16 who had social ages of over four years, 10 were in the home group. The children in this latter category were able to care for themselves at the toilet, wash themselves, dress themselves, print simple words, and play simple table games. Scale scores can be converted into a social age which is standardised for normal children, thus providing a reference point against which to a assess the develoipment of the severely mentally handicapped child. A social quotient can be calculated from the social age in exactly the same way as IQ is calculated, by dividing the social age by the child's chronological age and multiplying by 100. SQs of 100 indicate average social development for any given age and those below 100 indicate below average achievement.

Table 4.3: Social Quotient (derived from Vineland Social Maturity Scale)

Social Quotient	Home	Admissions	Total
<10	4 (9%)	18 (39%)	22 (24%)
11-20	7 (15%)	14 (29%)	21 (23%)
21-30	14 (29%)	3 (7%)	17 (19%)
31-40	8 (17%)	2 (4%)	10 (11%)
41-50	2 (4%)	7 (15%)	9 (10%)
>50	11 (24%)	2 (4%)	13 (14%)
Total (100%)	46	46	92

Table 4.3 shows the social quotients of the children in the home and admissions groups. In many respects the social quotient is more meaningful than the social age, since it provides a measure of the discrepancy between the child's actual achievement and what parents might

have expected from a normal child. Of the children who were awaiting admission, 70 per cent had social quotients of below 20 compared with only 24 per cent of the home group. Such social quotients indicated that their social ages were less than one fifth of their chronological ages, so that a child of 15 would have a social age of less than 3 years. Of the children in the home group, 24 per cent had SQs of above 50, although in most cases their intelligence quotients were below 50. Thus the level of social development of these children was considerably in excess of their intellectual achievements. Whilst the overall pattern of differences between the home and admissions group in the children's level of development is clear, it should be borne in mind that there were nine children in the admissions group who had social quotients of over 40 and, conversely, that there were eleven children in the home group with social quotients of below 20. Thus, the child's level of development was by no means the only factor involved in the decision to seek long-term institutional care.

Behaviour Problems

In addition to the many questions concerning the child's developmental level, mothers were asked about a wide range of potentially problematic behaviours. Up to a certain point, behaviour such as destructiveness, temper tantrums, hyperactivity, etc. is inversely related to the degree of disability, i.e. the more disabled the child the less likely he or she is to manifest such behavioural problems. The most severe problems tend to be presented by more able children, since many of the profoundly handicapped are incapable of such behaviour, simply because they are immobile. Nevertheless, Table 4.4. shows that a consistently higher level of behaviour disorders was found among the children awaiting admission than among those in the home group. A child was recorded as presenting a marked problem in a particular area of behaviour only when the mother reported that he or she behaved in this way always or frequently and that this constituted a problem for herself in particular and the family in general. Thus Janet, who had a tendency to spend periods of time screaming, was classified as a minor problem since her mother reported that she could usually be distracted without much effort. Susan's temper tantrums, on the other hand, which occurred two or three times every day and which often had a disruptive effect on other members of the family were recorded as a marked problem.

For many of the families in the admissions group, behaviour problems were a much more important factor in the decision to seek long-term care than the child's overall level of development. It is diffi-

Table 4.4: Behaviour Problems

	Home N = 46 (100%)	Admissions N = 46 (100%)	Total N = 46 (100%)
Destructiveness			
Marked problems	19 (41%)	26 (56%)	45 (49%)
Minor or no problems	27 (59%)	20 (44%)	47 (51%)
Screaming			
Marked problems	12 (26%)	23 (50%)	35 (38%)
Minor or no problems	34 (74%)	23 (50%)	57 (62%)
Temper Tantrums			
Marked problems	18 (39%)	26 (56%)	44 (48%)
Minor or no problems	28 (61%)	20 (44%)	48 (53%)
Hyperactivity			
Hyperactive	30 (65%)	30 (65%)	60 (65%)
Not overactive	16 (35%)	16 (35%)	32 (35%)
Behaviour in public places			
Marked problems	7 (15%)	20 (44%)	27 (29%)
Minor or no problems	39 (85%)	26 (56%)	65 (71%)
Difficulties with other children			
Marked problems	12 (26%)	16 (35%)	28 (30%)
Minor or no problems	29 (63%)	11 (24%)	40 (44%)
Does not play with other children	5 (11%)	19 (41%)	24 (26%)
Aggressive behaviour			
Marked problems	3 (7%)	7 (15%)	10 (11%)
Minor or no problems	43 (94%)	39 (85%)	82 (89%)
Rebellious behaviour			
Marked problems	5 (11%)	10 (22%)	15 (16%)
Minor or no problems	41 (89%)	36 (78%)	77 (84%)
Pestering for attention			
Marked problems	15 (33%)	18 (39%)	33 (36%)
Minor or no problems	31 (67%)	28 (61%)	59 (64%)

cult for parents of normal children to comprehend what these mothers meant when they reported a severe behaviour problem. Mary, who was awaiting admission, engaged her mother in a constant battle:

I can't think of anything at all that is easy with Mary, not even going for a ride in the car. We have to strap her to the front seat and she'll pull my hair and punch me. Her new habit is throwing her legs over my arm when I'm driving. We can't go anywhere in public like restaurants or shopping with her. She just sits on the floor screaming and kicking. If you let go she will grab any article in the shop and put it in her mouth. When she goes to bed at 8.30 p.m. she will bang on the window and stamp on the dressing table until 11 o'clock. We have been on holiday with 2 friends but even four adults cannot manage her.

The term 'behaviour problem' takes on a new significance in the light of such descriptions. The interviewers were often amazed at how families managed to cope at all under such circumstances.

The differences between the home and admissions groups in the proportions of children who presented marked behaviour problems were greatest in respect of behaviour which was likely to have an impact on people outside the immediate family. Of the 27 children who behaved badly in public places, such as in shops and on buses, 20 were awaiting admission to residential care. Parents either had to cope with obvious social disapproval whenever they took the child out, or they had to restrict severely their activities as a family. Similarly, of those children whose level of development was sufficient to enable them to play with other children, 29 per cent of the home group created problems compared with 43 per cent of the admissions group. It seemed that the effect of the child's behaviour on people outside the immediate family was at least as important as how the child behaved at home. The social stigma of a child who behaves badly in public may be as difficult to manage as one who is constantly destructive at home, although in some instances behaviour problems at home had effects outside the home. Michael's mother referred to his violent behaviour at home which also had effects outside the home:

> He has splints on his arms now to stop him bending them, but at one time he used to batter himself. He damaged his face and head and made himself black and blue. This caused people at the shops to accuse me of baby battering. They wouldn't believe that he had done it to himself. They used to say horrible things to me.

Just as the signficance of disabilities, such as incontinence or immobility, was dependent upon the age of the handicapped child, so the importance attached to behaviour problems was very much dependent on age and level of social development. Not only did children awaiting admission present more behaviour problems than those at home, but these were also concentrated more heavily in the higher age groups. There were 16 children in the admissions group who presented five or more of the behavioural problems listed in Table 4.3 and who were over eight years old. In contrast, the home group contained only four children in this category. Difficult behaviour became progressively more difficult to manage as the child grew older and developed a higher level of social maturity. The most difficult to manage were teenage children who were relatively independent. They combined physical strength with an ability to thwart any attempt to control their behaviour and an awareness of the effects it had on other people. One child in the admissions group had a passion for breaking windows and light bulbs. He could always find something to throw and could hit a light bulb from a distance of 15 ft. His mother found it virtually impossible to prevent him from doing this. She kept a supply of light bulbs in the house and called in a glazier to replace broken windows.

Summary

The data available on the handicapped chldren indicates that, in comparison with children in the home group, those awaiting admission to long-term care:

1. Were generally older.
2. Had slightly more problems with physical health.
3. Were more likely to suffer major functional incapacities.
4. Were less responsive to affection and were less likely to engage in social communication.
5. Required much closer supervision.
6. Were less socially mature and had much lower social quotients.
7. Were more likely to present major behavioural problems.

It is clear from the data presented so far that children awaiting admission to long-term care tended to be profoundly handicapped and/or behaviour disordered. They presented both practical and behavioural management problems, and families had to cope with these both inside and outside the home. However, it should be noted that although this review of the handicapped children has stressed the greater severity of problems experineced by parents of children in the admissions group, some parents of children not awaiting admission also experienced similar problems. The selection of children for long-term care is obviously related more than anything else to the nature of the problems presented by the children. But although the disabilities and behaviour of the child are important elements in the equation leading to residential care, many other factors are involved, some of which might be more emenable to change than those discussed so far.

Matching Like with Like

The relationship between family factors, felt needs, resources and levels of support received on the one hand, and the decision to seek long-term care for the handicapped child on the other, was the central concern of this study. Since the child's age and level of development clearly plays such an important part in the decision to seek long-term care, some allowance had to be made in subsequent analyses, which compared the home and admissions groups, for the differences between the children in the two groups. A matching procedure was therefore devised which made the two groups more comparable in terms of the difficulties presented by the handicapped child.

Each child from the home group was matched with one from the admissions group on the basis of age and social quotient. Age matching was carried out to within one year and social quotient to within 5 points. Since the differences between the home and admissions groups in terms of the child's age and social quotient were considerable, this second matching procedure considerably reduced the numbers available for further comparative analysis of the groups. The original total of 120 families was reduced to 60 for these analyses. However, where analyses in subsequent chapters are not concerned with a comparison of the home and admissions groups, tables refer to the total sample of 120 families.

The Families

As has already been noted, the basic unit of social structure in our society is the nuclear family and it is therefore within the family that the mentally handicapped child receives community care. However, the point has already been made that it is insufficient to identify the family as the unit of care. The division of labour within families means that the burden of care is not shared equally between different family members. In fact, mothers are the principal agents of care in the community, so community care usually means care by the mother.

The demands made on the mother by the presence of a severely mentally handicapped child, and how these are met, must be considered in the context of all demands which compete for her time. The extent of these demands and the resources, human and material, which she can call on to meet them vary greatly. Thus, the composition of the family, the definition of familial roles, the material conditions, the attitudes and expectations of the mothers and other family members, and the level of contact with people outside the family all contribute to the equation of needs and resources. Later chapters will consider the way in

which domestic tasks were allocated within families and the extent to
which outsiders, including the welfare services, contributed resources,
but before this is done the mothers and their families will be described.
The families are characterised in terms of the demands they made on
the mothers' resources and the resources, human and material, which
they contributed towards the meeting of all contingencies.

The Mothers

Comparing the 60 mothers in the matched samples, mothers of children
in the admissions group tended to be younger than those in the home
group. Of the former, 57 per cent were under 40 years of age compared with 70 per cent of admissions group mothers, although of the
five mothers who were over 50 years of age, only one was in the home
group. This suggests that decisions to seek long-term care were more
likely to be taken by mothers who were either relatively young or
relatively old when the handicapped child was born. Although the
numbers are small, the tendency for younger mothers to seek long-term
care may reflect a tendency for younger women to reject the traditional definition of their role within the family, and to see their lives in
broader terms than the continuing care of a severely mentally handicapped child. The importance of such changes in attitudes for the
decision to seek long-term care will be discussed in more detail later.

Mothers were asked about their current state of physical and mental
health, any illness or disability which constituted a problem for them
being recorded, whether or not treatment had been sought or obtained.
Most physical health problems reported fell into two broad categories,
general debility and chronic conditions which limited performance. The
former included being generally rundown, suffering from frequent
colds or lacking energy, whilst the latter included chronic bronchitis,
rheumatism and back problems. Assessment was based solely on what
the mothers reported, and whilst such an assessment may not describe
their objective state of health, it seemed more important to know how
the mothers felt about their health rather than how the doctors would
classify it.

The constant care necessary for many severely handicapped children
frequently has damaging effects on the health of the mother. Of all
mothers interviewed, 40 per cent reported some problem with their
physical health, but in spite of their younger age, problems were more
common among admissions group mothers than among those in the
home group. More than half of the former reported health problems
compared with less than a third of the latter. All six of the mothers who

reported a chronic condition which limited performance were among the admissions group.

Whilst problems falling under the heading of general debility constitute one factor among many others which might be taken into account in the decision as to whether to seek long-term care for the handicapped child, chronic conditions which limit the mother's capacity to carry out routine domestic tasks are more likely to have critical importance in the decision, since they have an obvious and long-term impact on the ability of the mother to continue caring for her handicapped child. The care and management of such a child in a house not adapted for the difficulties can become virtually impossible when the mother finds her own abilities severely impaired by poor health.

The strains experienced by mothers were not limited to their physical health. Problems of one sort of another with mental health were reported by 72 per cent of mothers, and these were divided into complaints for which the mothers had received no treatment and those for which they had received treatment in the past year. Forty-five per cent reported problems for which they had not sought any treatment, referring to a tendency to get nervy, on edge or depressed. As in the case of physical health, admissions group mothers were more likely to report problems than those in the home group (77 per cent compared with 67 per cent). In addition to this, they were also more likely to have received treatment for these problems, 33 per cent of admissions group mothers having had treatment for bad nerves or depression in the previous year, compared with 20 per cent of home group mothers. In some families the physical and psychological strains of caring for a handicapped child took a great toll on the health of the parents. Andrew was 12 years old, profoundly handicapped and awaiting admission to hospital. His mother described the strain and its effect on her own and her husband's health:

> I can't live like I should and the anxiety of seeing him in these fits is terrible. You feel helpless because you can't help the child. Sometimes I feel like a prisoner within these four walls. Sometimes you are up in the night with him. If I have lost sleep I am grumpy the next day. I am always getting colds and flu because I am so rundown. My husband got a hernia and two slipped discs through lifting Andrew. After tea you feel done in, tired out. There's been times when I have nearly been round the bend.

Mothers who have sought help from their general practitioners seemed to have received little in the way of effective treatment, support or even sympathy. Doctors had not, in general, mobilised the sort of support services which might have alleviated some of the health problems. Most mothers who had received treatment for mental health problems had been given tranquilisers or anti-depressants which did nothing to tackle the causes of the problems and frequently produced side effects, which mothers felt were worse than the original problem. Other doctors had offered no help whatsoever: 'I've been to the doctor but he wouldn't give me anything for my nerves. He said I must control myself and it's no good to take drugs.'

The health of many mothers might have been improved had they not been imprisoned in their own homes. For those who were fortunate enough to be able to go out to work, to be able to go out in an evening or to have a little free time to themselves at weekends, these things provided a life line to the outside world. However, 60% per cent of mothers did not go out to work at all, 40 per cent were unable to get out in an evening and 90 per cent had no free time to themselves at weekends. The importance of such activities in terms of the maintenance of good mental health has been highlighted in a recent study by Brown of depression amongst women.[4] Most of the mothers who did go out to work were only able to work part time and had to choose jobs which would allow them to be free during the school holidays. There was no appreciable difference between admissions group mothers and home group mothers in the proportions who were able to go out to work. Similarly the restrictions on opportunities for recreational activities applied equally to both groups.

Not surprisingly many mothers felt that they wanted to go out to work and that they ought to be able to enjoy at least some free time away from their handicapped child. Sixty-one per cent said that they would like to go out to work or, if they were already working, would like to work for longer hours. Most wanted to work not only for economic reasons, although the additional income would have been useful, but also because going out to work would have provided a degree of social contact which was otherwise unavailable. Although there was little difference between admissions group and home group mothers in the proportions already working, considerably more of the former wished to go out to work or work longer hours (Table 4.5). More than two-thirds of admissions group mothers wanted to work, compared with half those in the home group.

For many mothers evenings out were so rare they constituted an event which had to be planned well ahead and which was often trau-

Table 4.5: Would You Like to Go Out to Work/Work Full Time?[a]

	Yes	No	Total (100%)
Home	14 (54%)	12 (46%)	26
Admissions	20 (69%)	9 (31%)	29
Total	34 (62%)	21 (38%)	55

[a]Five mothers already held full-time jobs

matic because of the fear that something would go wrong. The following comment was characteristic of many mothers' feelings about leaving their handicapped child: 'I couldn't leave him with anyone. There's no one really knows him well enough. If we went out I would never stop worrying till I got back.'

Table 4.6: Would You Like to Go Out More?

	Yes	No	Total (100%)
Home	11 (37%)	19 (63%)	30
Admissions	23 (77%)	7 (23%)	30
Total	34 (57%)	26 (43%)	60

Nevertheless, many felt that something could have been done which would have enabled them to lead more satisfactory social lives. Dissatisfaction with their existing social lives and opportunities in recreation was much more common among mothers whose child was awaiting admission than among the home group mothers (Table 4.6). Of admissions group mothers, 77 per cent wanted to go out more in the evenings. Similarly, when mothers were asked whether they would like more time for personal recreation, as opposed to family activities, at weekends, it was the admissions group mothers who expressed more dissatisfaction. Of these mothers, 90 per cent wanted more time to themselves compared with 53 per cent of those in the home group (Table 4.7).

The consistently high proportion of mothers who expressed dissatisfaction with the opportunities available to pursue activities outside the family should provide those responsible for the planning of community services for the mentally handicapped and their families with food for thought. Existing services are based on the assumption that mothers are prepared to care for their handicapped child to the exclusion of most other activities. Many of the mothers interviewed for this study were

Table 4.7: Would You Like More Time to Yourself at Weekends?

	Yes	No	Total (100%)
Home	16 (53%)	14 (47%)	30
Admissions	27 (90%)	3 (10%)	30
Total	43 (72%)	17 (28%)	60

beginning to challenge this assumption in that they were not prepared to accept being unable to go out to work or to go out in the evenings. The fact that mothers whose child was awaiting admission were more likely than home group mothers to express these feelings reflects the inadequacy of community support services. They were faced with a choice of either continuing to devote their lives to a handicapped child or freeing themselves completely of the burden (and rewards) by seeking long-term care. There seemed to be no middle course available which would have enabled them to pursue activities outside the family and the home without having to seek long-term care for the handicapped child.

Mothers Alone

Although, as will be illustrated in later chapters, many fathers contributed little to the domestic routine they were, nevertheless, the principal source of support — and sometimes the only source — available to most mothers. One might have expected that single-parent families with a severely mentally handicapped child would face particularly difficult problems and would therefore be more likely to seek long-term care for the child. In fact, of the nine one-parent families in the matched groups, seven were in the home group. Thus, at least for these mothers, the fathers' absence, for whatever reason, did not appear to have made the difference between being able to support their handicapped children at home and being forced to seek long-term care. Unfortunately, information was not available from the survey concerning the reasons for the fathers' absence from home or how this affected the mothers' ability to cope with the situation. It is possible that in some families the relationship between the mother and handicapped child was made easier when the father was not present, since, from a purely practical point of view, the absence of the father can mean less work for the mother to do. It was not uncommon in families where the father was present for the mother to be expected to care for both the handicapped child and her husband, with little or no support. From an emotional and psychological point of view, the absence of the father may have meant that there were fewer demands on the mother's resources. In some families the presence of the handicapped child and the relationship between the mother and child may have created conflicts between the parents which were partly responsible for the father's departure. However, it should be noted that the predominance of single-parent families in the home group as compared to the admissions group is at odds with the findings of other studies of families with a mentally handicapped child.[5] A probable explanation for the disagreement between the findings of this study and those of other studies is that there have been changes in recent years in attitudes towards one-parent families. Single parenthood and illegitimacy no longer carry the social stigma which they did 20 years ago. Along with changes in the atttitudes of society at large have come changes in the attitudes and practices of the professions. Whereas in the past doctors and social workers tended to regard the departure of the father as sufficient reason for admission to long-term care, they are now more inclined to regard this as only one factor among many which must be taken into consideration.

The Fathers

Among the majority of families where the father was present their ages were similar to those of their wives, although slightly older. Of particular interest in the information collected about fathers was their employment, both in terms of whether they were in employment and if so what jobs they did. There was little difference between the home and admissions groups in the proportion of fathers in full-time employment, but the total of nine (18 per cent) who were not in employment was higher than might have been expected. No distinction was made between the registered unemployed and the sick, but in 1975, when the interviews were conducted, unemployment was rising. However, the economic activity rate for males between 25 and 60 years of age, was still well over 90 per cent for the country as a whole. The lower rate of economic activity among fathers in the study may reflect, in some cases, a tendency not to seek employment because of the additional support they were able to provide when not working. It is unlikely that fathers had actually given up jobs in order to help their wives but it is possible that some fathers, when they became unemployed, did not actively seek a new job.

Details of fathers' occupations, or last occupations for those not employed, provided the basis for an analysis of the relationships between social class and the decision to seek long-term care (Table 4.8).

There was, in fact, no clear pattern, although the numbers involved were very small. A higher proportion of families whose child was awaiting admission had fathers in non-manual occupations, but this probably only reflects the varying social class composition of the areas from which the samples were drawn. The home group was drawn from a predominantly lower social class inner city area, whereas the other samples included more families living in the outer city suburban areas, which had a higher proportion of residents in non-manual occupations. On the basis of the data available, it seems unlikely that social class is related to the decision to seek long-term care and this finding is in accordance with those of Tizard and Grad and Bailey.[6]

Table 4.8: Social Class (OPCS Classification of Occupations 1970)[a]

	I	II	IIInm	IIIm	IV	V	Total (100%)
Home	1 (5%)	0	1 (5%)	8 (38%)	6 (29%)	5 (24%)	21
Admissions	0	5 (19%)	0	9 (35%)	6 (23%)	6 (23%)	26
Total	1 (2%)	5 (11%)	1 (2%)	17 (36%)	12 (26%)	11 (23%)	47

[a]Insufficient information was available for 13 families

Mothers were asked about their husband's state of physical health and, although the fathers themselves might have reported more problems had they been asked, the level of problems was very low when compared to the problems that mothers reported for themselves. Seventy-four per cent of home group fathers and 71 per cent of those in the admissions group had no problems with their physical health, which suggests that the physical health of fathers is largely irrelevant to decisions relating to long-term care. Differences between the groups in the reported state of mental health of the fathers followed the same pattern as the mothers, fathers of children in the admissions group experiencing more problems than those in the home group. However, these differences were negligible when compared to the difference between the fathers and the mothers, only 18 per cent of the former experiencing mental health problems compared with 72 per cent of the latter. Whilst it is possible that the number of fathers suffering mental health problems was under-estimated, the figure of 18 per cent who experienced current problems with mental health was very close to the 14 per cent suffering from nerves, depression or irritability found by Dunnell and Cartwright among men as a whole. However, the 72 per cent of mothers reporting problems is more than two and a half times the figure obtained by the same authors for women in general.[7] The psychological burdens of caring for a handicapped child seem to fall very heavily on the mothers.

Siblings of the Handicapped Child

At different stages in the family cycle the influence of other children in the family on the balance between needs and resources changes. As children become older, the demands they place on other family members decline and in many families they begin to contribute resources. Their need for physical care and attention, in particular, reduces quite rapidly after the child starts school. At the same time, children gradually develop the ability, if not the inclination, to participate in domestic chores and the care of younger siblings. Thus the structure of families with a severely mentally handicapped child can be a very important influence on the extent to which parents are able to meet the demands of family life. It was expected that families in the admissions group would tend to be larger than those in the home group, to have more younger children and to experience more problems with the siblings of the handicapped child, thus creating a different balance between needs and resources. In the event, these patterns were not evident for the groups as a whole, although there were a few families in the admissions group in which problems experienced with other children constituted an important factor in the decison to seek long-term care.

Table 4.9: Number of Other Children

	0	1	2	3	>3	Total (100%)
Home	3 (10%)	4 (13%)	9 (30%)	4 (13%)	10 (33%)	30
Admissions	0	10 (33%)	9 (30%)	3 (10%)	8 (27%)	30
Total	3	14 (23%)	18 (31%)	7 (12%)	18 (30%)	60

Differences in family size were relatively small, although families in the home group had slightly more children than those in the admissions group (Table 4.9). The mean number of children (including the handicapped child) in the home group was 4.07 compared with 3.73 for the admissions group. This difference was not a consequence of variations in the ages of mothers in the groups, since families of admissions group mothers were smaller for all maternal ages. It is more likely that variations in family size related to the attitudes referred to previously in the discussion of the occupational and recreational aspirations of mothers. Mothers in the home group tended to define their roles more in family terms (including having larger families) whereas those in the admissions group tended to seek satisfaction in activities which did not necessarily involve their families.

Simple comparisons of the sizes of the families can, however, be misleading, since some of the children had already left home at the time of the interview and the ages of those remaining at home ranged from one year through to children in their twenties and thirties. The provision of practical and material support by children was dependent upon their age and whether or not they lived in the family home, although the presence of older children was no guarantee of any support. Comparison of home and admissions groups in terms of the number of children living at home revealed the same pattern as for total family size, the mean for the former being 3.43 (including the handicapped child) and for the latter 3.00. The ages of children are an important factor in determining whether they constitute a drain on or a contribution to the family's resources. It is likely that children under seven years of age are on balance a drain on resources and those over twelve years of age are, at least potentially, able to contribute resources. There was, in the event, little variation between the groups in the age distribution of children. Although slightly more families in the home group contained children over 16 years of age living at home, slightly more families in the admissions group had children in the 12- to 16-year age group. At the other end of the spectrum, admissions group families contained more younger children; there were six families with pre-school children in the home group and nine in the admissions group. This probably reflects the larger number of younger mothers in the admissions group. Nevertheless, they were faced with the double burden of a handicapped child and the full-time care of one or more other dependent children at home. Mrs Evans (home group) had two pre-school children as well as her handicapped child: 'When I have to go shopping it is terrible with the three little ones. I've no trolley now so I have to wait till my sister comes at the weekend. She minds the children and I go shopping.'

Mothers were asked whether they experienced any problems with their other children. Whether or not they reported any problems was dependent on whether they perceived their children's behaviour as problematic. The fact that very few mothers did report problems with other children, rather than indicating that there were no difficulties, suggests that what problems did occur paled into insignificance beside the problems of caring for a severely mentally handicapped child. The number of home group mothers who reported problems of any sort was similar to the number in the admissions group, but the type of problem reported by mothers in the two groups was different. Six siblings of children awaiting admissions were severely mentally handicapped, educationally subnormal or suffering from long-term physical health problems compared with two in the home group. Most of the problems reported by mothers in the home group were less specific and were usually seen as only temporary. The existence of long-term problems in a sibling of the handicapped child, as well as increasing the burden of care on the mother, may also have helped to legitimate the parents' request for long-term care. It enabled the parents themselves to feel easier in their own minds about taking the decision, and it was an important factor in legitimating the request in the eyes of doctors and social workers.

Material Conditions

Though one might expect poorer families to be more likely to seek long long-term care for a handicapped child, evidence from other studies is conflicting. The study by Tizard and Grad, carried out in the 1950s, reported no difference in material conditions between a home group and an institution group, but more recent studies by Bailey and Jaehnig have reported that poorer families were more likely to seek institutional care.[8] An accurate assessment of the balance between material needs and resources would require detailed information about family income and expenditure, and the collection of such data would have been difficult and time-consuming. However, information was collected on total income, the possession of various consumer durables and the type of housing in which families lived. According to these criteria there were no gross differences in living standards between families in the home and admissions groups.

Table 4.10: Total Weekly Income[a]

	≤£40	£41-£50	£51-£60	£61-£70	>£70	Total (100%)
Home	5 (19%)	5 (29%)	7 (26%)	9 (33%)	1 (4%)	27
Admissions	6 (22%)	4 (15%)	5 (19%)	8 (30%)	4 (15%)	27
Total	11 (20.4)	9 (16.7)	12 (22.2)	17 (31.5)	5 (9.3)	54

[a]Insufficient information was available for six families

Information on total family income was collected for 54 of the 60 families in the matched groups (Table 4.10). Five home group families had incomes of less than £40 per week compared with six in the admissions group, but there were one and four families respectively with incomes of over £70 per week. Since admissions group families were drawn from a wider and on average more affluent geographical area, the data suggest that total family income was unrelated to the decision to seek long-term care. There was, however, a tendency for fathers in the admissions group to have higher incomes than those in the home group. Of the former, 21 per cent had incomes of over £55 per week compared with 5 per cent of the latter. The only other important source of income in the majority of cases was the Constant Attendance Allowance (CAA) which, at the time the interviews were carried out, was £9.20 per week. Of all families, 85 per cent were receiving a full allowance, but of the nine who had no income from this source or only received a partial allowance, six were in the home group. Whilst the CAA has provided a valuable source of income to many families with a handicapped child, failure to inform families of their rights and variations in the interpretation of ambiguous regulations have caused many difficulties. Among those who were receiving the allowance, there were many who had learned of their right to claim only through talking to other parents, some of whom had endured a long struggle to obtain the allowance. In families where the handicapped child was able to go for regular periods of short-term care, family finances were often disrupted because payment of the allowance was stopped whilst the child was away from home. Such bureaucratic regulations caused some hardship, made many parents feel they were accepting charity and, in my view, were unproductive, since any savings achieved must have been largely offset by the costs of administration.

Table 4.11: Consumer Durables

	Home N = 30 (100%)	Admissions N = 30 (100%)
Radio	30 (100%)	28 (93%)
Television	30 (100%)	30 (100%)
Record player	24 (80%)	21 (70%)
Washing machine	27 (90%)	25 (73%)
Fridge	23 (77%)	22 (73%)
Clothes drier	6 (20%)	4 (13%)
Vacuum cleaner	23 (77%)	23 (77%)
Car	14 (47%)	11 (37%)

The other method used to describe the material circumstances of families was to look at the number of families possessing each of a basic range of consumer durables, which most modern households might consider as necessitites (Table 4.11), and the type of housing in which they lived. All families owned or rented a television set which, for many, was a vital means of keeping the handicapped child occupied. The 50 per cent of families who owned, or had the use of, a car found that it opened up a whole new range of activities. Although the majority of families possessed the basic consumer durables there were some who lacked such essentials as washing machines, fridges and vacuum cleaners, the majority of these being in the admissions group. Whilst such domestic appliances might have been regarded as luxuries 20 years ago, most households today regard them as essential. For the family with a handicapped child there can be no question that they are necessary to ensure a satisfactory quality of life. There were no major differences between the home and admissions groups in the type of housing in which they lived, but more of the latter lacked certain basic amenities. A total of twelve families had no inside toilet and six had no bathroom. These conditions are, unfortunately, not uncommon in the Manchester conurbation, but the fact that these families cared for a severely mentally handicapped child in these houses is appalling.

Conclusions

This chapter has attempted to outline the characteristics of the mentally handicapped children, those who cared for them and their living conditions. It is already apparent that the relationship between conditions existing in the family and the decision to seek long-term care of the handicapped child is highly complex. There is no simple connection between the availability of human and material resources in the family and whether or not the child can be coped with at home. In some respects, families whose child was not awaiting admission were worse off then those in the admissions group, but in other respects they appeared to be better off. In most cases, however, the differences were marginal. Of far greater importance were the problems experienced by mothers and how they felt about their situation. More mothers in the admissions group were in poor physical and mental health and more expressed dissatisfaction with various aspects of their lives. Subsequent chapters in this book deal almost exclusively with the experiences of the mothers and their needs for additional support. Those responsible for providing services to the mentally handicapped and their families must become increasingly aware of the importance of how mothers respond to the situations in which they find themselves.

5 THE DAILY ROUTINE

In order to begin to understand family life with a severely mentally handicapped child, it is essential to look at the mundane household activities that constitute the daily routine; this chapter tries to convey how caring for a handicapped child dominated the mothers' lives. Other members of the family were affected but nobody else experienced the total domination that was felt by the mothers. This was community care in practice, and the effects it had on the lives of the people who did the caring are revealed in the mothers' own descriptions of their day-to-day experiences. The ways in which child care and household tasks were allocated and dealt with are described in quantitative terms as is the level of support mothers received with different tasks. A discussion of who provided support and who might have done more to help is left until later chapters as is a discussion of the mothers' felt needs for additional support and the services that might have been provided to alleviate the problems. The domestic routine is, for the purposes of analysis, divided into a number of physical child care, child minding and housework tasks. This is necessary in order to do more than describe the circumstances of each individual family, but it has the disadvantage that it removes these tasks from their overall context. Such analyses do not enable the reader to obtain an impression of the day-to-day lives of families with a severely mentally handicapped child. The extent of the child's influence on the domestic routine varied greatly from one family to another. In order to convey an impression of how the children affected family life this chapter begins with detailed descriptions of three families and their very different experiences of caring for a handicapped child.

Three Examples

Sheila

This was a profoundly handicapped twelve-year-old girl with a level of social and intellectual functioning which was below that achieved by the average one-year-old child. She lived with her parents and her elder brother and sister (16 and 18 respectively) in a well maintained owner-occupier terraced house with a small garden situated in a quiet street. The house was modernised and Sheila had her own bedroom. It was, however, rather small and, as is true of many older houses, the stairs were steep and difficult to manage with a non-ambulant child. Sheila was unable to walk at all, although she could shuffle and crawl, she required somebody to feed her, could only manage a liquid diet and wore nappies day and night, since she was doubly incontinent. Thus she was totally dependent for physical care on the other members of the family. In addition to this, she appeared not to respond to any form of communication, had a tendency to bang her head repeatedly on the sides of her cot or on the floor and frequently slept very badly at night. Not surprisingly the family's domestic routine tended to revolve around Sheila and her requirements.

She usually woke in the morning at about 8.00 a.m. and was carried downstairs by her father before he left for work at about 8.15 a.m. Although her mother could just about manage to carry her up and down stairs this was becoming increasingly difficult. Between 8.15 a.m. and 9.10 a.m. her mother was more or less fully occupied in feeding, washing and dressing Sheila before the ambulance arrived to take her to the special school. She often refused to eat any breakfast at first but could usually be persuaded to eat something. Washing and dressing Sheila was not easy at the best of times, but was made particularly difficult when she was unco-operative. Being co-operative meant a passive acceptance of her mother's attempts to wash and dress her, but when she became difficult in a morning she tried to scratch or bite anybody who attempted to dress her. One way or another Sheila had to be ready by the time the ambulance called, and her mother was then able to get on with general housework. The fact that she wore nappies and required a complete change of clothing twice a day meant that her mother had to wash clothes at least three times a week. She was, however, more fortunate than some mothers who faced similar problems in that she had an automatic washing machine. At about mid-morning she usually had to postpone the remainder of the housework in order to visit her elderly father who lived in the same neighbourhood. After checking that he was all right and doing some cleaning and shopping for him, she was able to do her own shopping and return home in time to prepare lunch for her husband. Any remaining housework and the preparation of the evening meal had to be completed by about 4.00 p.m. when the ambulance brought Sheila home from school. Although Sheila would usually play with her toys until the family gathered for tea at about 6.00 p.m., she could not be left in a room alone for more than about one minute. She usually wanted something to eat at the same time as the rest of the family, but this required one person to feed her whilst saving their own meal. For the rest of the evening she would play as before under close supervision and was usually ready for bed between 9 and 10 p.m., although she often did not go to sleep until midnight. She was carried upstairs to bed by her father who, because she slept poorly, went to bed at about the same time so that he could be in the room with her until she went to sleep. During the night he would get out of bed every two to three hours to see that Sheila was not banging her head and had not become uncovered. Weekends were similar except that Sheila had to be occupied throughout the day, but since the whole family was usually at home, the tasks of playing with her, feeding her, dressing her, changing her, etc. could be shared. School holidays, however, were much more difficult since, although the routine was essentially the same as at weekends, the burden of care fell very heavily on her mother. The older children were not around and her father was working. For about four weeks of the summer holiday (her father arranged two weeks holiday to coincide with the school holidays) her mother had to look after Sheila all day in addition to performing all the usual household tasks and helping her invalid father.

Paul

This was a hyperactive fourteen-year-old whose mental and social capacities were similar to those of the average four-year-old child. He was fully ambulant, fully continent and capable of performing most self-care tasks with only minimal supervision. However, these abilities were combined with an over-active temperament, very little sense of danger, a desire to wander and an ability to overcome most obstacles that might be placed in his way to prevent his wandering. His older brothers and sisters had all left home, leaving only Paul and his elderly parents in a small rented terraced house. His father was an invalid and had been unable to work for a number of years and his mother had suffered periods of ill health during the previous two years.

There was no regular time at which the day could be said to begin, since this was largely dependent on what time Paul decided to get up, which varied between 5.00 a.m. and 9.00 a.m. One parent had to get up with him in the morning, usually his mother, since he could not be left alone for fear that he would injure himself or manage to get out of the house (he once went to school at 6.00 a.m. dressed only in jumper and socks before his parents realised he had left). From the time he got up to the time he was ready for school somebody had to be with him in order to keep him out of mischief. Dressing, feeding and washing him had to be accomplished during this time and, although he was quite capable of performing these tasks for himself, he often refused, which resulted in a long verbal battle since he was becoming too big for force to be effective. The school bus called at a collection point not far from Paul's home, but his mother had to wait anything from five minutes to half an hour for the bus to arrive. She found it a great relief every day when Paul eventually went to school. However, she found that the time he was away — between 9.30 a.m. in the morning and 3.30 p.m. in the afternoon — only provided just sufficient time for her to get through the usual domestic chores. Paul's over-active behaviour meant that he was extremely hard on clothes and created a great deal of extra housework. The housework and the preparation of the evening meal had to be finished by the time Paul returned at 3.30 p.m. If the weather was reasonable his mother would take him to the local park in order to try and work off some of his seemingly limitless energy, other-wise he would have to be occupied at home which meant more or less constant supervision. The evenings provided some respite as Paul was prepared to sit and watch television, although he could not be persuaded to go to bed until 11 or 12 o'clock.

When he did eventually go to bed he insisted on sleeping with his mother and, even so, there was no guarantee that he would stay asleep. It was not uncommon for his mother to wake and find that Paul was downstairs playing records at 2.00 a.m. One consequence of Paul's behaviour at night was that his parents had not had a satisfactory sexual relationship for a number of years. Without the relief provided by Paul's attendance at school, weekends and school holidays could be torture. His mother felt that she was incapable of physically keeping pace with Paul's needs, her invalid husband's needs and the housework. Neverthe-less, she managed to get by with the assistance of substantial periods of short-term care for Paul during the school holidays.

Graham

This child presented a sharp contrast to the two already described. He was nine years old and lived with his family in a modernised three-bedroomed council house. Like Paul he was fully ambulant and capable of basic physical self-care with only minimal supervision but, unlike Paul, he presented no behaviour problems. His mental and social capacities were similar to those of a normal five- to five-and-a-half-year-old. He had two older brothers and one twin brother and seemed to fit into the normal pattern of family life as the youngest child in the family. The family's daily routine appeared to be adapted to Graham's needs but to no greater extent than one might expect in a family with a young child. He rose in a morning at the same time as the other children and was quite capable of getting himself ready for school with minimal supervision. The school bus called for him at a local collection point at about 8.45 a.m., and his mother was able to work between 9.00 a.m. and 1.00 p.m. in a local supermarket. She was able to complete her housework after returning from work and before Graham came home from school. The amount of housework was not excessive since the children, including Graham, helped to keep things tidy. The family usually had tea between 5 and 6.00 p.m., after which Graham would play with his brothers and their friends either indoors or outdoors. He went to bed at about 9.00 p.m., the same time as his twin brother. Weekends and holidays were similar except that Graham played out more. Holidays presented a bit of a problem but his mother had been able to continue working because Graham's 16-year-old brother was able to keep an eye on him during the school holidays.

The contrast between Sheila, Paul and Graham in terms of the influence they had on the daily routines of their respective families illustrates the difficulties involved in referring to such families as an homogenous group. Each family was unique in terms of the problems they faced and the ways in which they coped with them. However, in order to go beyond the presentation of case histories on each individual family situation, it is necessary to identify problems common to all families with a handicapped child and to analyse ways of dealing with these in a framework which is applicable to most families. For the purpose of this study, 15 categories of child care and household tasks were used to classify the basic daily activities which constitute the core of the daily routine. The child-care items were oriented towards the specific problems of caring for a handicapped child and were divided into two sections: physical child care and child minding. However, the questions were not addressed exclusively to the problems of caring for the handicapped child, since to have done so would have ignored the demands made by other children.

Physical aspects of child care

Mothers were asked whether any of their children required assistance or close supervision with each of the tasks listed in Table 5.1. If at least one child in the family required help or close supervision with a particular task, the mother was then asked who usually did the task and whether or not anybody else helped. Individuals were classified as participants if they usually undertook the task or shared it more or less equally with one or more others, and as helpers if they provided only occasional support without undertaking responsibility for the task. In general the mothers themselves drew the distinction between participants and helpers. Up to three participants and four helpers could be recorded for each task.

Table 5.1: Physical Care of Children

	Not applicable	Mother	Mother & helper	Shared	Total (100%)
		Who usually does this?			
Dressing children					
Home	1 (3%)	9 (30%)	16 (53%)	4 (13%)	30
Admissions	0	13 (43%)	13 (43%)	4 (13%)	30
Total	1 (2%)	22 (37%)	29 (48%)	8 (13%)	60
Washing children					
Home	1 (3%)	18 (60%)	7 (23%)	4 (13%)	30
Admissions	0	11 (37%)	17 (57%)	2 (7%)	30
Total	1 (2%)	29 (48%)	24 (40%)	6 (10%)	60
Nappies					
Home	16 (53%)	9 (30%)	3 (10%)	2 (7%)	30
Admissions	14 (47%)	11 (37%)	3 (10%)	2 (7%)	30
Total	30 (50%)	20 (33.3%)	6 (10%)	4 (7%)	60
Toiletting					
Home	10 (33%)	8 (27%)	7 (23%)	5 (17%)	30
Admissions	12 (40%)	6 (20%)	10 (33%)	2 (7%)	30
Total	22 (37%)	14 (23%)	17 (28%)	7 (12%) q	60
Feeding children					
Home	4 (13%)	7 (23%)	13 (43%)	6 (20%)	30
Admissions	9 (30%)	7 (23%)	8 (27%)	6 (20%)	30
Total	13 (22%)	14 (23%)	21 (35%)	12 (20%)	60
Lifting and carrying					
Home	19 (63%)	3 (10%)	6 (20%)	2 (7%)	30
Admissions	18 (60%)	2 (7%)	5 (17%)	5 (17%)	30
Total	37 (62%)	5 (8%)	11 (18%)	7 (28%)	60

Table 5.1 shows the number of families in the matched home and admissions groups who had children who required help or close supervision in each of six aspects of physical child care. For those whose children did require help or supervision, Table 5.1 shows the extent to which the mothers received support from any source. Virtually all families had children who required washing or dressing and a large majority had a child who required some supervision at meal times and with toiletting. Half had children who wore nappies and 38 per cent had

a child who required lifting and carrying. For those physical child-care tasks that did require performing on a daily basis, it was notable how few mothers were able to share the responsibility for the tasks. Although there were differences between mothers in the home group and those in the admissions groups, these were small and followed no particular pattern. The numbers of mothers in either group who received significant levels of support with physical child care were very small, but some tasks attracted more support than others. The pattern of support in relation to specific tasks reflects a traditional interpretation of conjugal roles, in that certain tasks were performed almost exclusively by the mothers whilst others were much more likely to be shared with other family members. The extent to which particular child-care tasks were viewed as maternal role obligations varied according to the nature of the task. Those which required most physical contact with the child were most likely to be performed by the mother with no support from anybody else. In two-thirds of the families who had a child wearing nappies the mother received no help at all with nappy changing, but in families where children required feeding or closely supervising at meal times only 30 per cent of mothers received no help with this. Similarly, whilst half of the mothers received no help with washing children (another task which necessitated close physical contact) only 37 per cent received no help with dressing. Close physical contact with children is traditionally regarded as part of the maternal role and most fathers take little part in the physical care of babies and very young children. In these families with a handicapped child this definition of roles extended to children who were chronologically and physically much older. The lower the level of physical contact necessary for a particular task the more likely it was that responsibility would be shared or at least support provided. The only task which did not fit into this pattern was lifting and carrying the child. For families in which at least one child was non-ambulant only 22 per cent of mothers received no support. This reflected the fact that a number of the non-ambulant children were quite old and therefore very heavy. It was hardly surprising that other family members were often involved with lifting and carrying such children, since mothers were often unable to manage alone. Nevertheless, some of those who were managing without help had to lift children of nine and ten years of age.

Catering for the handicapped child's basic physical needs sometimes presented enormous problems. Mothers were asked what aspects of caring for him or her they found most difficult and the problems of physical care often featured in their accounts:

> she wets the sheets nearly every night. Also you have to sit and feed
> her. Carrying her is getting very difficult. She is 11 years old now and
> and she is heavier than she looks. Bathing is difficult because it is
> hard to get her in the bath and then she won't sit up. She won't rest
> her hands on the bath so it's hard for me to wash her and to wash
> her hair. If my husband is in he does the carrying but he is not
> always here.

This child was in the home group but such accounts of the problems of
physical care were more characteristic of mothers whose child was
awaiting admission. Jane was on a waiting list for hospital and her
mother said:

> It's most distressing and she wets a lot. If I am on my own I have to
> change her and change the bed and turn her. She is a big girl and
> quite heavy. She is nearly fifteen and its getting very hard to lift her.
> She keeps wetting herself when she is in a fit and I have to change
> everything, even the pillowcases. It is very hard to cope.

However, there were a number of mothers, particularly in the home
group, who dismissed these problems. For example, Gillian was ten
years old, non-ambulant and doubly incontinent but her mother said:
'It is the incontinence and the feeding that are most difficult but I have
had her so long that I have just got used to it.'

Three mothers of children in the admissions group referred specifically to a problem which was not dealt with directly in the questionnaire, that of menstruation. They were finding the problems of dealing
with menstruation in their teenage handicapped daughters a great
strain. Mrs Harris, whose daughter Susan was referred to the study by a
social worker, explained these particular problems:

> Her periods are the biggest problem. She is forever going to the toilet
> and she sits there screaming for ten minutes. I don't know why and
> I've got to stand with her all the time. At period time she is worse.
> She still expects me to go with her and change her. It is very difficult
> for her to understand and it's very embarrassing for me with three
> boys in the house. She goes to the toilet more when she has got a
> period and constantly wants clean towels. I can be in the middle of
> cooking dinner and she wants me to take her to the toilet and change

her.

It is clear from these examples, that the physical care of the handicapped child, particularly the older child, can have an enormous impact on the daily routine of the family and the mother in particular. In general, mothers of younger children and older children who were ambulant and continent did not perceive physical care as such a problem. In relation to the amount of physical care necessary these children were usually sufficiently close to normal expectations not to be classified by their mothers as problems in this respect.

Minding Children

Despite claims that the nuclear family in modern society has abdicated responsibility for the care and upbringing of children and that these functions have largely been taken over by the state, families do in fact retain overall responsibility for the well-being of children. Whilst the educational system plays an important role in their upbringing, most children of school age spend only about one seventh of their lives in school. Thus the responsibility borne by the parents for the child's welfare far outweighs that borne by the state, and, in almost every instance, the responsibility borne by the mother far outweighs that borne by any other individual. This allocation of responsibility for child rearing, whether or not it is desirable, is accepted by most parents as an integral part of family life. However, the severely mentally handicapped child often far exceeds normal expectations in terms of the expenditure of time and energy necessary to fulfil parental responsibilities. He or she does not make the normal progression towards independence which is expected of children. All of the handicapped children in the families in the matched home and admissions groups, even those with relatively high levels of development, required close supervision during their waking hours and in some cases even when they were asleep.

Table 5.2 divides the children's time spent at home into four periods; after school and before bed time, night time, weekends and school holidays. Each of these was a period during which somebody had to be responsible for the care and supervision of the handicapped child. As in respect of physical child care, it was the mothers who were usually responsible for providing this supervision, although the number of mothers receiving support varied greatly. The extent to which they were wholly responsible for minding children depended largely on the availability of other family members capable of relieving them of the burden. Table 5.2. shows that although only 13 per cent of mothers

Table 5.2: Minding Children

	Who usually does this?			
	Mother alone	Mother with help	Shared	Total (100%)
After school				
Home	14 (47%)	15 (50%)	1 (3%)	30
Admissions	15 (50%)	7 (23%)	8 (27%)	30
Total	29 (48%)	22 (37%)	9 (15%)	60
Weekends				
Home	6 (20%)	11 (37%)	13 (43%)	30
Weekends	5 (17%)	7 (23%)	18 (60%)	30
Total	11 (18%)	18 (30%)	31 (52%)	60
School holidays				
Home	17 (57%)	10 (33%)	3 (10%)	30
Admissions	18 (60%)	5 (17%)	7 (23%)	30
Total	35 (58%)	15 (25%)	10 (17%)	60
Baby-sitting				
Home	4 (13%)	7 (23%)	19 (63%)	30
Admissions	4 (13%)	5 (17%)	21 (70%)	30
Total	8 (13%)	12 (20%)	40 (67%)	60

received no help with baby sitting and only 18 per cent received no help with minding children at weekends, 58 per cent had nobody to relieve them in the day time during school holidays and 48 per cent had nobody to help when the children returned home from school every day. In the light of the fact that most families spend their weekends as a group, it might be regarded as slightly surprising that only half of the mothers reported that they were able to share child minding at weekends, and eleven mothers received no help whatsoever. Similarly, one might have expected that virtually all families would be able to share the responsibility for baby sitting between family members. In the event, only two-thirds of mothers reported that this task was shared and, in many cases, this simply meant that both mother and father stayed at home. As far as the mothers were concerned this meant that they were still as closely tied to the child at home as ever.

The school holidays and the periods after school and before the evening meal were times at which, in most families, the mother was the only responsible person able to look after the children. In the case of normal children the amount of attention required tends to decline steadily once he or she begins attending school, and by the time most children reach the age of seven or eight years, the number of hours during which mothers are required to provide direct supervision are few.

For many severely mentally handicapped children, however, the amount of supervision necessary remains as much, and often more, than would be given to a normal 0-3-year-old child. In most of the families in this study there was no prospect of an end to this state of affairs. Although, as was seen in the previous chapter, some of the handicapped children had achieved a considerable degree of independence in self-care, this was usually not accompanied by a corresponding development in other spheres which would have reduced the necessity for close supervision. Fully mobile, toilet-trained children who were able to dress, wash and feed themselves, often required very close supervision, because they had no understanding of simple dangers, were apt to wander off, or were likely to become aggressive or destructive. Para-doxically, some of the most severely handicapped children were less of a problem from this point of view because they were immobile and therefore not capable of putting themselves in danger when left alone. For most of the 35 mothers who were solely responsible for minding children during the school holidays this meant being unable to leave the handicapped child alone for more than two or three minutes at a time. The same was true for the 29 mothers who received no help with children after school and the 11 who received no help at weekends. It is difficult for most people who have not experienced such problems to comprehend what life for these mothers was like. They were tied to the care of a highly dependent child for 24 hours each day with no prospect of relief other than that provided by the child's attendance at school.

Differences between the home and admissions groups in the propor-tions of mothers receiving support with child minding were very small. However, of those who did receive some support, mothers of children awaiting admission seemed somewhat more likely to share the activity rather than only to receive help with tasks which remained their responsibility. Thus, only one of the sixteen home group mothers who received help with children after school described herself as sharing responsibility, compared with eight of the fifteen whose child was awaiting admission. Similarly, in the school holidays, three mothers in the home group shared the job of minding children compared with seven of those in the admissions group. In most families where responsi-bility for minding children was shared it was the fathers who provided the support for their wives. It is possible that in families where the father was drawn into the tasks of child care, through taking responsibility for child minding, the mothers' definitions of the situa-tion as overwhelming or impossible to cope with were more likely to receive legitimation. When the father had to take some responsibility for the problems he was more likely to regard them as serious and to feel that something must be done. Thus the decision to seek long-term care was more likely to be legitimated within the family. Mothers who carried the burden alone sometimes blamed themselves if they felt unable to cope, and thus saw residential care as an admission of failure rather than as a reasonable solution to an intolerable situation.

When mothers were asked what were the main problems in looking after their handicapped child, the most commonly mentioned difficulty was the constant attention required. This was often mentioned in a general way, but there were specific times when it became particularly burdensome. Many, including Mrs Jones who was in the home group, made specific reference to the school holidays:

> When he's at home it is awkward. He can't play in the back yard because the steps are too steep. I can't get anything done because he is always running around. If he sits down you've got to sit with him. It's the constant attention. Just the little things in themselves but he always needs watching.

Another mother in the home group described similar problems but interpreted them differently:

> She's not really bad. I have just got to watch her all the time. It is at night more than anything. Once she fell down the stairs. You've just got to keep your eye on her all the time, but she's no trouble really.

The problems that these two mothers exprienced were in many ways very similar, but the way they felt about these problems was very different. In the second example, the mother had resigned herself to the need to provide constant attention and the resulting domination of her own life. The mother of Mary Dean, in the admissions group, provided yet another interpretation of the problem of providing constant attention. This was a more middle-class family and Mrs Dean's description of problems tended to emphasise the importance of keeping Mary stimulated. She also made specific reference to the problem of finding suitable baby-sitters as did many mothers:

> Keeping her stimulated is a problem. Well it means you've more or less got to be keeping her attention all the time. I mean the normal looking after Mary is just a part of living. I don't class that as anything now. It is just part of having Mary. But children like this

deteriorate rapidly if they are not stimulated. It is just that at times you are tired yourself, I'm 46 not 26. I just haven't got the physical strength. I think that this happens to all Mums who have this type of child. It's very difficult to get baby-sitters. Your social life goes by the board. The people you can leave children like Mary with are few and far between and we can never go out together. Either I go or my husband goes.

Many parents were concerned to provide the best possible learning environment for their handicapped child and were prepared to devote considerable time and effort to provide the necessary stimulation. Others felt that they would like to do more, but they were not sure how best to help him or her to learn. There was often, as will be evident in a later chapter, a lack of communication between the home and the school, which meant that parents were not aware of the sort of things their child was doing at school, and were therefore unable to reinforce these activities at home. This certainly did nothing to alleviate the problems presented to many families by school holidays, when mothers and children suffered unrelieved boredom and social isolation for long periods. The six-week summer holiday was particularly difficult for many mothers. Sharon's mother felt that she could cope during term time but the school holidays imposed a very great strain on her:

It's in the holidays that I feel it most. I usually get very depressed, in fact I am dreading this next fortnight when they are on holiday. I think its just the fact that you can't go anywhere. For a week she seems to be alright but then she seems to get bored and you get more of the screaming then. You have no time to yourself. When they are at school you do get a bit of time but when they're on holiday there's just no time.

Housework

A mistake that is sometimes made when considering the problems of caring for a severely mentally handicapped child in the family is to emphasise the problems of child care to the exclusion of other aspects of the daily domestic routine. Cooking, ironing, washing and shopping all have to be carried out by somebody, and it is important, in establishing how the burden of community care is distributed, to look specifically at these tasks. It has been noted in the previous two sections of this chapter that large proportions of mothers received no help with the various aspects of child care. Unfortunately, this lack of support was not compensated for by an increased level of help with basic household chores. In all five household tasks about which mothers were asked, most undertook the responsibility for the task themselves and many received no assistance from anybody (Table 5.3). There were, however, marked differences between tasks in the proportions of mothers who received help. Only 28 per cent received any help at all with washing and ironing clothes, but 78 per cent received some help with washing dishes, laying the table, etc. There was an obvious hierarchy in which tasks such as washing clothes and cooking were clearly designated as maternal role obligations, whereas washing dishes and shopping were much less clearly defined obligations and were therefore activities in which other family members were much more likely to play a part. It is worth noting, however, that even with washing dishes and shopping, 52 per cent and 78 per cent respectively of mothers bore the main responsibility for the task. The numbers who were fortunate enough to be able to hand over complete responsibility for individual household tasks was very small. Among the 60 mothers in the matched home and admissions groups there were only 10 who were completely relieved of washing dishes and 7 who were completely relieved of shopping. Although there has been a tendency in recent years to stress the increasing equality of husband and wife in marriage today, as compared with the nineteenth and early twentieth centuries, it is clear that housework remains very much the wife's responsibility in most families. A discussion of who provided the support that was available to the mothers and different patterns of conjugal role organisation will be left until the next chapter. For the time being the most important point is that the majority of mothers carried a very heavy burden with very little support.

As in relation to child care tasks, differences between mothers in the home group and those in the admissions group in relation to the amount of support received with housework were small. In general, more mothers whose child was awaiting admission were receiving some support except with washing dishes and shopping. Also more of these mothers shared tasks with somebody or were completely relieved of certain tasks. For example, nine of the ten mothers who were relieved of the responsibility of washing dishes were in the admissions group. Thus, in relation to housework, what differences there were between the mothers in the matched groups favoured those whose handicapped child was awaiting admission.

The mothers' descriptions of the problems they experienced in relation to child care have already touched on the impact that the

Table 5.3: Housework

| | Who usually does this? | | | | |
	Mother alone	Mother plus help	Shared	Other	Total (100%)
Washing clothes					
Home	25 (83%)	5 (17%)	0	0	30
Admissions	18 (60%)	8 (27%)	3 (5%)	1 (3%)	30
Total	43 (72%)	13 (22%)	3 (5%)	1 (2%)	60
Cooking					
Home	21 (70%)	8 (27%)	1 (3%)	0	30
Admissions	16 (53%)	11 (37%)	2 (7%)	1 (3%)	30
Total	37 (62%)	19 (32%)	3 (5%)	1 (2%)	60
Cleaning					
Home	15 (50%)	13 (43%)	2 (7%)	0	30
Admissions	11 (37%)	13 (43%)	5 (17%)	1 (3%)	30
Total	26 (43%)	26 (43%)	7 (12%)	1 (2%)	60
Shopping					
Home	7 (23%)	19 (63%)	2 (7%)	2 (7%)	30
Admissions	8 (27%)	13 (43%)	4 (13%)	5 (17%)	30
Total	15 (25%)	32 (53%)	6 (10%)	7 (12%)	60
Washing dishes					
Home	5 (17%)	14 (47%)	10 (33%)	1 (3%)	30
Admissions	8 (2-%)	4 (13%)	9 (30%)	9 (30%)	30
Total	13 (22%)	18 (30%)	19 (32%)	10 (17%)	60

handicapped child often had on housework. There were two principal effects on the day-to-day running of the home which varied in relative importance, depending on the particular circumstances, but the effect of both was to increase the burden of ordinary household chores. First, the handicapped child tended to create extra work, and secondly, many of the children prevented mothers from doing housework by demanding constant attention. Alan Small's mother emphasised the extra work created and the additional expense this involved, rather than the fact that he prevented her from getting on with the housework:

I have to clean his room every day with Dettol. It always has the smell of wee no matter how hard I scrub it. The expense of keeping up with all these things is so great. Dettol is 30p. a bottle. I have terrific problems with clothes washing, etc. I am always in trouble with the Social Security for spending too much on heating, but I have to bath him three times a day and do the washing every day.

On the other hand Mrs Marshall found that, although her daughter Jane did not create much additional housework, she often prevented her from doing routine household tasks:

> It's not that she makes a lot of work like some of them do, she just won't let me get on with things. When she's off school I have to do the cleaning and washing after she's gone to bed. It is all right for a week or so but after that I start to get so tired. Then I get grumpy and that just makes things worse.

But such reorganisation of the household routine to fit in with the handicapped child was not always class as a problem. John Fairbrother was not awaiting admission and his mother said:

> I don't class John as a rod for my back, he is not a problem to me. He just needs me and that's what I am here for. He's no problem to any of us. You have to do things to suit John. I do all my washing and shopping while John is at school so I can leave the weekend free for him. I have to give him a lot of my time that's all.

Finally, there were those whose handicapped child prevented them from doing the housework and created large amounts of additional work. Andrea Beamish was in this category:

> It's a very long day for me. I am not married and I lost my mother last year. I get very lonely. She never sits still so I am on the go all the time. When she's at home I couldn't possibly do any housework or cleaning or go upstairs to make beds or anything. I have to spend every minute with her. There's just no let up and there's so much washing all the time. She is constantly wet from dribbling. She rolls in the dirt and everything needs constant washing.

Conclusions

The severely mentally handicapped children in the matched groups referred to in this chapter made a great impact on the daily routines of their families and particularly their mothers. This was true whether or not the child was awaiting admission to long-term residential care. On the one hand they created direct demands on the mothers' resources which were often very difficult to meet and, on the other, they often prevented them from giving attention to competing demands. Almost all mothers found that the handicapped child in one way or another dominated their daily routine. Most resented this to a greater or lesser degree, although there were a few in the home group who, whilst recognising the impact the child had, did not see this as a problem.

In all aspects of the daily routine which were considered, the majority of mothers in both the home and admissions group bore the main responsibility for carrying out whatever tasks were necessary. The numbers who received support varied according to the nature of the task, which reflected the extent, with regard to both child care and household tasks, to which these were defined as maternal role obligations. Differences between the home and admissions groups in the proportions of mothers receiving support were small. More mothers of children in the admissions group received support with more tasks and they were also more likely to share responsibility for the tasks rather than receiving help. Although such differences were small they are interesting in that they contradict the initial hypothesis that home group mothers would be likely to receive more support in their daily routine than those in the admissions group. It would be dangerous, however, to interpret this finding as an indication that the provision of domestic support is irrelevant to the decision to seek long-term care. The level of support received by these mothers was, in most cases, so abysmally low that it had little bearing on the decision. Had support been available at a level which made a significant impact on the daily domestic routine, the story might have been very different.

6 WHO HELPS?

The previous chapter concluded that community care does not mean care by the community, nor does it mean care by the family, it means maternal care with varying but generally low levels of support from others. In most cases mothers carried the burden of child care and housework with little support from their families, relatives, friends and neighbours. A recent study of mothers showed that this pattern was very much the norm for all families.[1] The mothers of mentally handicapped children in this study faced special problems but they did not have special resources at their disposal to deal with these problems. Nevertheless, it was apparent from the data presented in the last chapter that there were many instances of support from these informal sources which, if they did not exactly amount to a sharing of the burden in most cases, at least eased the load on many mothers. In order to develop a comprehensive picture of community care, it is important to look closely at the contributions of different individuals. It is easy to create a picture of what community care *should* be like, involving shared responsibilities in the family, supportive neighbourhoods and close-knit kinship networks, but it is less easy to describe the actuality and to suggest ways in which support might be increased. If analyses are to be useful as guides to the professions working with the mentally handicapped and their families and to policy-makers taking decisions about future services, they must provide details of exactly what support is being provided and by whom. Only in this way is it possible to assess what resources are at present available to families and consider how these can be linked to a service network designed to complement informal networks.

This chapter deals with the support provided by other family members and by relatives, friends and neighbours. Attention is focused on those individuals who provided most support for mothers in the daily routine of caring for the handicapped child and fulfilling their other obligations. Consequently, most attention is devoted to the role played by fathers, since they constituted the greatest single source of support. The reasons why some fathers contributed more than others and the ways in which their contributions might have been increased are discussed. After fathers, the siblings of the handicapped children were the next most important source of support, but their contribution was small even in relation to that of their fathers. The reasons for this generally low level of support, the factors which seemed to affect whether or not siblings helped and the potential for developing support from this source are considered in this chapter. Finally, support from outside the nuclear family is considered. Interestingly, the findings of this study contrast sharply with those of some others, where much higher levels of support inside and outside the family were reported. The reasons for these apparently contradictory findings are discussed, as is the potential for developing greater community support. Since the focus in this chapter is upon a description of community support for the majority of mothers with a severely mentally handicapped child, rather than on the question of the relationship between levels of support and decisions to seek long-term residential care, the tables presented, in the main, refer to all the families in the samples rather than to the groups matched on the basis of the child's age and social quotient.

Fathers

Although in most families the father was the principal source of support available, the level and nature of the help he provided varied greatly. In some families he contributed nothing to either child care or housework, whilst at the other extreme, there were fathers who participated equally in almost all tasks. Linda's father was at one extreme and his wife said:

> she depends on me you know. Well I think a woman should do these jobs, but when he was off work he wouldn't even change her nappy, even if it was only wet he wouldn't change her. He said: 'You see to her, I'm not doing that.' Linda hasn't made any difference to him. He's always gone out. I'm the one who's had her, he doesn't do anything.

On the other hand, Sheila's father shared most jobs when he was at home, his wife said:

> I feel that parents should combine and each do whatever happens to need doing. For instance, changing nappies and feeding children, that's a woman's job technically, but John helps me with that. We share the jobs. He will cook a meal if necessary and he always washes the dishes.

As will become evident later in this discussion, although these two examples represent extremes of the spectrum, Linda's father was far more typical than Sheila's. It was noticeable that even Sheila's mother, when describing her husband's contribution, indicated that she considered the jobs to be technically hers. She implied that her husband's contribution was a response to special problems and special circumstances. All of these families of course faced special problems by definition and, before analysing the contributions that fathers made to the solution of these problems, it is worth placing this in context by briefly referring to what is known about the organisation of the domestic routine in families who do not face such problems.

The sociology of housework and child care is a relatively neglected area, in spite of the fact that a large proportion of the population spend most of their lives engaged in rearing children and looking after the home. However, in recent years the attention that sociologists have devoted to these subjects has thrown some light on the contributions of fathers to the daily domestic routine in families without the additional burden of a handicapped child. The data collected by different researchers is variable in quality and the level of participation reported for fathers seems to depend, to a considerable extent, on the way in which questions were asked. Young and Wilmott, in their study of families, reported that 72 per cent of the fathers performed tasks other than washing dishes at least once a week.[2] Such a finding is unremarkable, but what is remarkable is that the study is entitled *The Symmetrical Family*. This data could be used to support the conclusion that the majority of fathers contribute, at least minimally, to the domestic routine, but not, as Young and Wilmott attempt to do, to conclude that there is increasing symmetry in role relationships in the nuclear family. They made no distinction between shared responsibility for tasks and merely providing a helping hand, and their data failed to distinguish between fathers who went shopping once a week and those who cooked, cleaned, washed and looked after the children. At the other extreme, Ann Oakley asked, for specific child care and household tasks, how often the husband had carried them out over a defined period of time, and concluded that 60 per cent of fathers in her sample had a low level of participation in housework and 45 per cent in child care.[3] However, even Oakley's classifications of high and low levels of involvement were only relative to other fathers in the sample. Thus what was termed a high level of support did not necessarily indicate an equal sharing of tasks. The evidence suggests that the majority of fathers make at least a minimal contribution to the domestic routine but that only a small proportion contribute to an extent that would justify the description of *shared* child care and housework.

The two studies mentioned above clearly show that the way in which the problem is posed and the nature of questions asked about the domestic division of labour in the family have a considerable effect on the findings and the conclusions which are drawn from them. In this study it was not feasible to collect diaries recording the actual performance of domestic tasks over a period of time, but it was considered essential to ask about specific tasks and who actually did them. Mothers were asked who *usually* did each particular job rather than who did it yesterday or last week. The answers were recorded in the form of named participants (i.e. those who usually did the job) and named supporters or helpers (i.e. those who only helped, rather than sharing the responsibility). Any individual, inside or outside the family, could be classified in either category provided that he or she met the necessary criteria.

Table 6.1: Father's Participation in Child Care and Household Tasks

Task	Participant	Support Helper	No support	Total (100%)
Physical child care[a]				
Dressing	17 (17%)	30 (30%)	54 (54%)	101
Washing	21 (21%)	29 (29%)	51 (51%)	101
Nappies	9 (14%)	17 (26%)	39 (60%)	65
Toiletting	11 (20%)	15 (27%)	29 (53%)	55
Feeding	20 (24%)	32 (39%)	31 (37%)	83
Lifting	30 (53%)	19 (33%)	8 (14%)	57
Minding children				
After school	15 (14%)	28 (27%)	62 (59%)	105
Weekends	51 (49%)	24 (23%)	30 (29%)	105
School holidays	7 (7%)	15 (14%)	83 (79%)	105
Baby sitting	71 (68%)	12 (11%)	22 (21%)	105
Household tasks				
Cleaning	10 (10%)	23 (22%)	72 (69%)	105
Cooking	7 (7%)	28 (27%)	70 (67%)	105
Washing dishes	33 (31%)	23 (22%)	49 (47%)	105
Washing clothes	3 (3%)	10 (10%)	92 (88%)	105
Shopping	24 (23%)	29 (28%)	52 (50%)	105

[a] Includes only those fathers who had a child who required the task performing or who required close supervision

Table 6.1 shows the proportions of fathers who provided support for their wives in each of 15 child care and household tasks. There were only two tasks in which more than half of the fathers were described as participating equally with their wives: lifting and carrying the child and baby-sitting. The former is a special case in that some of the non-ambulant handicapped children were too heavy for their mothers to lift without help. The father's help in lifting and carrying such children was not a reflection of a willingness to participate in child care but a practical necessity of daily living. The meaning of shared responsibility for baby-sitting is unclear, since it frequently meant merely that both parents were at home in an evening, although it was usually the mother who actually looked after the children. In general, fathers' participation in physical aspects of child care was dependent on the degree of physical contact necessary. Tasks such as changing nappies and bathing children required much closer physical contact than supervising dressing and helping at meal times. Of fathers who had an incontinent child, 60 per cent provided no assistance in changing nappies, but at the other end of the physical care spectrum, only 37 per cent gave no assistance with supervising children at meal times. Whether or not fathers spent any time minding children was clearly dependent on whether they were available when needed. Whilst 70 per cent and 73 per cent respectively, helped with baby sitting and looking after children at the weekends, only 41 per cent helped after school and 21 per cent during school holidays. Thus, it seemed that fathers were likely to be involved with minding children, even in families where they took no part in physical child care or housework. Diane's father would take no part in her physical care but his wife said: 'She thinks a lot of her Dad. I look after her but when he's here he will play with her. On Sunday he took her out at 2 o'clock and came back at 5 o'clock. That gave me a chance to get some housework done.' Oakley reported similar findings with respect to normal families, where fathers regarded it as part of their role to play with children but not to provide physical care.[4]

The level of fathers' participation in housework was generally lower than in child care, a finding which has been confirmed by other research workers looking at normal families. The only tasks in which a significant number of fathers participated, at a level approaching equality with their wives, were washing dishes and shopping. These were perhaps the least arduous of the tasks included in the questions. In many families this was the only concession to sexual equality in the home. Washing dishes was, in some families, regarded as a male responsibility:

Well, I will be fair. I've never washed a pot since I've been married — only a cup or something. After tea he always washes up. He always has done. When we were both working I used to get the tea but he used to wash up.

In this family, as in many others, this was where sexual equality ended, since the father provided no assistance with any of the other domestic tasks. In spite of the fact that many of the handicapped children created large amounts of extra washing, only 12 per cent of fathers provided any help at all with washing and ironing clothes.

An examination of the support provided by fathers in individual tasks, whilst useful in comparing levels of participation for different tasks, does not facilitate comparisons of overall levels of support provided by fathers in different families. A scoring system was devised in order to assess the overall contribution made by the fathers in different families and to assess their contribution to physical child care, child minding and housework. Construction of a score to reflect the overall level of support necessarily involves taking arbitrary decisions to convert essentially qualitative data into quantitative form, but only in this way is it possible to make comparisons based on an overall picture rather than treating individual items separately. It was clear from looking at the interview schedules that scores achieved by the fathers on the scale generally agreed with the interviewer's subjective assessments of their levels of participation in particular families. For each of the tasks, a score of 1 was given if he took responsibility or shared the responsibility, half if he helped and 0 if he provided no support. The scores for each item were then added and the result divided by the number of applicable tasks (e.g. if the handicapped child did not require lifting and was not wearing nappies the number of applicable tasks would be 13 rather than 15). Thus, for all tasks taken together, a score of 1 indicated maximum participation and, at the other extreme, 0 indicated that he provided no support at all. In the same way as a score for overall support was arrived at, scores for each of the three sections (physical child care, minding children and household tasks) were calculated. Only a quarter of fathers achieved a score of more than 0.5 taking all child care and housework tasks together (Table 6.2). The fact that most were in full-time employment limited the extent to which they could be expected to participate in the domestic routine, but there was no reason why all fathers could not have achieved a score of at least 0.5 by providing help with most tasks and participating equally in one or two. It is difficult to see why, from a practical point of view, virtually all fathers could not have shared with their wives minding children at weekends, baby-sitting, cleaning the house, washing dishes and shopping. The only tasks with which a large number of fathers might not have been able to help at all were minding children after school and during the school holidays. In order to justify assertions of equality in marriage, a large proportion of fathers would need to score at least 0.5 on the scale used, but in fact, three-quarters of this sample scored below that figure and a third provided only minimal support.

Table 6.2: Participation Scores of Fathers

Task area	Low 0-0.25	Medium 0.25-0.5	High 0.5-0.75	0.75-1	Total (100%)
Physical child care	44 (42%)	33 (31%)	15 (14%)	13 (12%)	105
Minding children	33 (31%)	40 (38%)	24 (23%)	8 (8%)	105
Household tasks	55 (52%)	39 (37%)	8 (8%)	3 (3%)	105
All tasks	35 (33%)	44 (42%)	23 (22%)	3 (3%)	105

It is difficult to make a comparison between these findings and those of studies that have looked at the domestic division of labour in ordinary families since, as mentioned above, different studies have used different methods of assessment. Some, such as those of Bott and Gavron have concentrated on what fathers would or should do (i.e. the normative aspects), rather than what they actually did on a day-to-day basis.[5] To ask what fathers should do with respect to the domestic routine may be useful in terms of understanding attitudes and accepted norms, but it is not possible to infer from answers to these questions what actually happens. Ann Oakley's study of housewives provides perhaps the best comparative standard, since she attempted to assess exactly what fathers did in respect of child care and housework. She reported that only 15 per cent of husbands had a high level of participation in housework and 25 per cent in child care.[6] However, she did not describe how her high and low levels of participation were arrived at, merely that high levels were relative to other fathers in the sample rather than to any absolute standard. Nevertheless, the pattern of fathers' participation reported by Oakley was broadly similar to that found in the present study. This suggests that fathers of severely mentally handicapped children adopted domestic roles which varied very little from the dominant cultural pattern.

Apart from the generally low level of participation of fathers in the domestic routine shown in Table 6.2, the other important finding is the fact that the extent of their involvement varied between the three different groups of tasks. Fathers were most likely to be involved in aspects of child care rather than housework and, within the general area of child care, rather more with minding children, particularly in the evenings and at weekends, that with the physical aspects of child care. This discrepancy between child-care roles and housework roles is very similar to that reported by Oakley. The considerable difference between the two areas can largely be explained through different attitudes to child care and housework as paternal role obligations. Within broad limits the role of the father in the day-to-day life of the family is socially prescribed. He is expected to play with children and take them out but not to change nappies and dress them or to wash clothes and cook meals. In most families this means that his role in child care increases as the child grows up, but in families with a severely mentally handicapped child this process either does not take place or is spread over a much longer period of time. In many cases the handicapped child does not develop sufficiently for the father to be able to play his usual role. Playing games in the park or taking children to the cinema are activities which might normally constitute part of the father's role but which, in a family with a severely mentally handicapped child, may be inappropriate. There was some evidence, however, to indicate that fathers of the most profoundly handicapped children adapted their roles to meet the requirements of the situation, in that more of them became involved in physical child care. Only 28 per cent of those whose child had a social quotient of below 10 had a low level of participation in physical child-care tasks compared with 57 per cent of those whose child had a social quotient of above 40, yet when all child care and household tasks were taken together, there was only a slight difference in the levels of participation of fathers with children at different ends of the spectrum. Thus it seemed that although the severity of the handicap did not affect the overall level of participation of the father, it affected the nature of the tasks in which he participated. Fathers of profoundly handicapped children had made some attempt to adapt their roles to the specific problems, although they might have done much more.

If the severity of the child's handicap had only a small effect on the fathers' level of participation, what other factors can be suggested to explain variations in the extent to which they were involved in the domestic routine? Some shared the burden of care with their wives, others contributed a significant amount of support but the majority failed to make more than a token contribution. It is important, from the point of view of developing family care in the community, to look at what factors might have explained the different levels of contribution by fathers. It was shown in the previous chapter that the overall level of support received by mothers was not related to whether or not the handicapped child was awaiting admission to long-term residential care. Similarly, there was little relationship between specific contributions made by fathers and whether or not the child was awaiting long-term care. More or less the same proportions in both the home and admissions groups had a high level of participation, although slightly more of the latter achieved a moderate level. As suggested in the previous chapter, a limited involvement in child care and housework on the part of the father might have resulted in the mother's problems being taken more seriously, therefore providing additional support for the decision to request long-term care.

Table 6.3: Fathers' Participation by Age

Participation (all tasks)	Fathers' age (yrs)			
	⩽ 30	31-40	> 40	Total
Low	7 (44%)	11 (24%)	17 (40%)	35 (33%)
Medium	7 (44%)	18 (39%)	19 (44%)	44 (42%)
High	2 (13%)	18 (37%)	7 (16%)	26 (25%)
Total (100%)	16	46	43	105

Other factors which might have been expected to influence the extent of fathers' participation were age, employment and social class. The relationship between fathers' age and the level of participation is shown in Table 6.3. Those under 30 years of age had the lowest level of participation followed by those over 40 years, but the difference between these two groups and the 31 to 40 age group is greater, although in all cases the numbers were small and conclusions must be tentative. It is possible that those in the 31 to 40 age group had a higher level of involvement in family affairs in general than either younger or older fathers. The children of those fathers who were under 30 years of age were more likely to be under school age and the families were smaller,since family building had in many cases not been completed. The nature and amount of work in the home during this period of the family cycle tends to result in a clearer definition of child care and housework as maternal responsibilities. This is combined with the fact that this period is one of considerable financial strain for most families, because the family increases in size and money has to be spent on the home and its contents. Thus it is likely that fathers in the under 30 age group were working longer hours and were therefore less available to participate in child care and housework. In the 30 to 40 age group the pressures on material resources tend to be less severe, the care of children involves tasks of a different nature, the children are older, but the overall level of work necessary in the home is greater because the family is larger. For these reasons one might expect fathers in this age group to have a higher level of participation, particularly in child care, whilst a decline in the level of participation of those in the higher age groups might be expected. Children are older and therefore expected to be less dependent. Also the attractions of family life may have worn thin and, whereas mothers are tied to their obligations, fathers are more able to choose their level of involvement. The fact that one of the children in each of the families in this study was severely handicapped and did not conform to expectations regarding independence, did not appear greatly to affect the pattern of participation of fathers. Finally, we may be seeing signs of changing attitudes towards the father's role in successive cohorts. Those fathers in the 31 to 40 age group may continue to have a higher level of particpation as they grow older, but it is impossible in a small cross-sectional study of this sort to show whether whether this process is actually taking place.

Table 6.4: Fathers' Participation by Employment

Participation (all tasks)	Fathers employment		
	Employed	Not employed	Total
Low	32 (35%)	3 (23%)	35 (33%)
Medium	40 (44%)	4 (31%)	44 (42%)
High	20 (22%)	6 (46%)	26 (25%)
Total (100%)	92	13	105

Table 6.4 shows the relationship between the level of participation and whether or not the father was in full-time employment. Not surprisingly, the level of participation of those not in employment was higher than the others, but the difference was much smaller than might have been expected if one assumed that the main reason for a low level of support was the fact that they had to go out to work and were therefore unable to perform many of the tasks. Nevertheless, 46 per cent of unemployed fathers had a high level of participation compared with only 22 per cent of those in employment. Although information on the reasons for fathers not working and the length of time that they had been out of work was not collected, it is possible that those with a

high level of participation were not keen to return to work. In other words, long-term unemployment is one possible strategy that families might adopt in order to deal with problems of providing care for a severely mentally handicapped child. Whether or not these fathers had stopped working in order to help in the home it is impossible to say, but it is likely that some had been incorporated in a more or less permanent way into the economy of the family, and that for them to go out to work again might have been seriously disruptive to the established pattern of organisation of family life. Finally, Table 6.5. shows the level of participation of the fathers from different social class backgrounds. The social class gradient in fathers' involvement in the domestic routine is similar to that observed by other researchers.[7] Those in the top three social classes had a higher level of participation than the others but, particularly in the high participation category, the difference was less than has been suggested by other authors. The tendency for higher social class fathers to be more involved in child care and housework reflects differing norms regarding paternal role obligations among different social groups and varying degrees of jointness in conjugal roles, as well as perhaps shorter or more flexible working hours. In the pilot interviews, which dealt with attitudes to conjugal roles in some detail, it was noticeable that, in the two families where the fathers had non-manual occupations, both parents stressed the fact that they shared domestic tasks. In contrast, families in social classes IV and V stressed a greater division of labour, although the difference in attitudes was not always reflected in the actual organisation of the domestic routine. However, it would be wrong to suggest that middle-class families were characterised by a pattern of joint congujal roles whereas working-class families were characterised by segregated conjugal roles. The patterns of conjugal roles in the families in this study could be said to have a greater or lesser degree of jointness in respect of domestic labour, reflected in the husband's level of participation, but to dichotomise them into joint or segregated would ignore the range of behaviour. It also might wrongly imply, in relation to those described as joint, a degree of sharing tasks which in fact existed only rarely.

In summary, it can be said that the father's role in the majority of families was much less than it might have been. There were indications as to why some fathers contributed more than the average and some less, but the inescapable conclusion is that most could have and should have done more to ease the burden on their wives. They were not very different from most ordinary fathers in the extent of their contribution,

Table 6.5: Fathers' Participation by Social Class

Participation (all tasks)	Father's social class			
	I, II, III non-manual	III manual	IV, V	Total
Low	2 (13%)	15 (42%)	15 (31%)	35 (33%)
Medium	8 (53%)	13 (36%)	21 (44%)	44 (42%)
High	5 (33%)	8 (22%)	12 (25%)	26 (25%)
Total (100%)	15	36	48	99

but the difficulties faced by their wives were much worse than those faced by most other mothers. By and large, both husbands and wives accepted the division of labour. The mothers did not expect more of their husbands and, although they often felt severely oppressed by the burdens of child care and housework, they did not usually blame this on their husbands. However, these comments should not be taken to imply that the status quo is inevitable or should be perpetuated. If fathers could be encouraged to play a bigger role in child care and housework this would result in a lessening of the burden carried by mothers, but the way in which this might be tackled requires careful consideration. The doctor, social worker, nurse or voluntary worker in close long-term contact with a family and its problems is in an ideal position to begin to suggest alternatives to the existing domestic division of labour. However, to suggest wholesale changes in the way husbands and wives organise their domestic routine would be impracticable and would, in most cases, be rejected, but by dealing with specific problems changes might be encouraged. Fathers were engaged in child minding activities more than other child-care or household tasks, but this was sometimes restricted because the handicapped child required physical care, e.g. changing nappies which the father could not or would not do. In addition, it appeared that some, although prepared to mind the handicapped child, did not know what to do with him or her. The father's role in the upbringing of normal children tends to mean he has little experience in the sort of play and learning activities appropriate to very young children. The severely mentally handicapped child often remains at this level, thus making it difficult for the father to become involved. Discussions between parents and professionals of these sorts of problems might reveal ways in which fathers might both increase their contribution and gain more satisfaction out of caring for their handicapped child. Their participation in routine household tasks might also be increased by tackling a specific problem. For example, in a family in which the handicapped child created large amounts of extra cleaning, the father might be persuaded to share in this task by discussing the problems with both parents and explaining how his help could ease the burden on his wife. But this sort of approach can only work if the professions working with families have continuing relationships with both parents and can, therefore, offer advice which takes account of all the circumstances.

The Children

As a source of support in the daily routine, next in importance to the fathers were the siblings of the handicapped child. Most of the research that has been conducted on the nature of child care and housework for families in general and families with a mentally handicapped member in particular has ignored the sometimes important role played by children or has only made passing reference to it. Ann Oakley, for example, devotes a whole chapter to a discussion of the division of labour between husbands and wives but makes no reference to the supportive role of children.[8] The role played by children in the care of their siblings and in housework, although much smaller than that played by their fathers, can nevertheless constitute an important factor in reducing the burden placed on the mother in some families. Clearly children constitute a drain on the physical, emotional and material resources of their parents during their early years, and in many cases continue to be a drain on resources until they leave home. However, they are also able to make a positive contribution to various aspects of the domestic routine from a relatively early age. Even five or six-year-old children can perform a useful service by playing with younger siblings, and as they become older there are numerous household tasks that they might participate in.

Table 6.6: Participation Scores of Children

Task areas	No support 0	Low 0.1	Medium 0.1-0.3	High 0.3	Total 100%
Physical child care	260 (74%)	18 (5%)	29 (8%)	44 (15%)	351
Minding children	26 (77%)	0	51 (15%)	32 (9%)	351
Household tasks	227 (65%)	32 (9%)	54 (15%)	28 (11%)	351
All tasks	195 (56%)	58 (17%)	57 (16%)	38 (11%)	351

Table 6.6 shows the contribution of children to child care and housework. The method of calculating scores for participation was the same

as that described for fathers in the previous section, but the categories of high, medium and low participation were much lower than those used for fathers, since most children made a small contribution. Because of the large proportion of children who provided no support, an additional category was included. Since all siblings of the handicapped children were included in the analysis, the number of children providing support does not represent the number of families in which support was available to the mother. In some families more than one child provided support whereas in others no support was available from children. Since children of all ages were included in Table 6.6, it is hardly surprising that the 'no support' column contains a large number of children, but it shoud be remembered that a total of 153 chidren were providing some support with child care and/or housework. This represents a very important resource available to at least some of the 120 mothers. Unlike their fathers the children were slightly more likely to help with household tasks than with child-care tasks and, within the category of child-care tasks, there was littler difference between physical care and child minding tasks. For example, 52 children helped with dressing the handicapped child, 29 helped with toiletting, 31 helped with minding during school holidays, and 53 helped with baby sitting. Among the range of household tasks considered there was only one in which more than 20 per cent of children provided some support. This was washing dishes which, interestingly, was the only household task with which a large proportion of fathers provided assistance.

Where an older child did help with child care and housework this could be an important source of support for the mother. Susan Johnson had a teenage brother and sister who could both be relied upon to help. Her brother would keep an eye on her while her mother went out to work and her sister contributed to the ordinary domestic routine. Mrs Johnson said:

> When the children get older, such as my girl, they should help. She helps me a lot with the housework. I think they should. When she gets married she's got to do it herself and she knows how to go about it. When she was at school she would watch Susan for two or three weeks in the summer holidays.

In some families the most important contribution of siblings was baby-sitting whilst the parents went out together in an evening. The most important criterion for the baby-sitter was that he or she should be very familar with the handicapped child and, therefore, older siblings were often the only people with whom the mothers felt happy about leaving the child. Mrs Marshall was able to leave her six-year-old mongol daughter with her twelve-year-old son:

> It's only recently that we've been able to get out in an evening, but it has made such a difference to me. A friend used to baby-sit occasionally for Jane but I never felt happy about leaving her. I was always worried that something might happen. It is different leaving her with Michael. He knows her as well as we do and I can rely on him to see that she's all right.

Whether or not children provided assistance with either child care or housework was related to their age and sex but not to whether or not their handicapped sibling was awaiting admission to long-term care. Not surprisingly, very few children under seven years of age were able to contribute anything. Slightly over half of the children in the 8-11 age group made some contribution to the domestic routine. Support rose to a peak in the 12-16 age group where three-quarters provided some assistance and almost a third had a relatively high level of participation. Among the 16+ age group the level of support dropped sharply as children found jobs and left home. Thus the greatest potential for support seems to be among the 12-16 age group, but within this group it is quite heavily concentrated among girls. Of the 38 children who provided a high level of support, 31 were girls. This difference between the contribution to the domestic routine of girls and boys suggests that the sexual division of labour in parental roles is in the process of being repeated in the next generation. One of the mothers said: 'Well, I think they should help. My children help me. They wipe the pots and do odd jobs like that. I think older children should muck in with the mother, especially girls anyway. I mean you don't expect a man to do it quite as much . . . '

The implications of these patterns of support for families with a severely mentally handicapped child are considerable. The size of the family reflects the nature of the tasks that have to be completed as part of the normal daily routine, but the age and sex structure of the family affects the extent to which mothers have to cope alone with the problems. Those mothers with daughters in the 12-16 age group were most likely to receive a significant amount of support from their children, but it must be remembered that the age structure of the family is constantly changing. The development of the family cycle means that there are periods in which children constitute only a drain on parental resources, periods in which they contribute resources and eventually a point is reached when, for most families, they constitute neither a drain nor a contribution to resources. The difference between the families in this study and normal families was the presence of a handicapped child who did not fit into the usual pattern. He or she usually remained dependent whilst the other children passed through the normal stages of development. Thus, mothers who may have relied on help from the child's older siblings found themselves worse off as they grew up and left home. There were a number of families in which teenage children were an important part of the routine and where mothers expressed doubt about how they would manage when these children left home. Of the 49 children who had left home, only 9 were still providing any support and 7 of these provided only minimal assistance. This should be weighed against the relatively high level of support provided by children in the 12-16 age group which is the period immediately prior to their leaving home.

The overall level of support provided by children was not related to the severity of their siblings' handicap. It was simlar in those families with a profoundly handicapped child and in those with a child approaching the educationally subnormal level. This may reflect a desire, on the part of the mothers, not to impose the burden of their handicapped child on the other children. Some said that they made every effort to ensure that the lives of their other children were not adversely affected. John made a great deal of extra housework but his mother said: 'Well my girls have never done anything like that. I thought I had enough of that. They have always had a kind of lady's life.'

It is difficult to know whether any changes are taking place in the domestic roles of children and whether, in the future, children will contribute more or less to the daily routine. However, a number of mothers did comment that they felt that children were becoming much more independent and were therefore less likely to participate in the home. This is certainly a view of young people which is conveyed by the media, but there is scant evidence to indicate whether or not it is true in practice. There were certainly a sufficient number of children in the present study who made valuable contributions to both child care and housework to at least reject the blanket assumption that all young people today are motivated purely by self-interest.

For the professions whose job it is to advise and support families with a handicapped member, this discussion of the role of children in the home underlines the importance of looking at the family as a whole and maintaining a long-term perspective. Children can be both a drain on resources and a contribution to them and the balance changes over time. They, like their fathers, could perhaps do more to help, both in caring for the handicapped child and helping with housework. Their contribution might not be a major one and is usually limited to a period of between five and ten years before they leave home. It can nevertheless be valuable, not just in terms of easing the burden, but in establishing a pattern of shared domestic responsibilities and familiarising more people with the problems of care. The social worker or community nurse should be aware of this potential and be able to suggest ways in which children might participate as they grow older. In addition, he or she should be aware of the short-term nature of any support provided by children, and therefore be prepared to suggest alternatives for when they leave home. These alternatives may be other informal sources or it may be necessary to replace the support of children with an additional service commitment, at least in the short-term.

Relatives, Friends and Neighbours

The theory of community care makes great play of the support derived from outside the nuclear family. The 1971 White Paper, *Better Services for the Mentally Handicapped*, in its general principles stated that 'understanding and help from friends and neighbours and from the community at large are needed to help the family maintain a normal social life and to give the handicapped member as nearly a normal life as his handicap or handicaps permit'.[9] There was, unfortunately, no further mention in the White Paper of what help might be provided by these people or how common in practice it was for families to receive this sort of help. There is a long tradition in sociology, philosophy and social administration of emphasising the importance of community and expressing concern at the supposed loss of community associated with industrial development. In post-war years the work of the Institute of Community Studies and, in particular, Young and Wilmott's *Family and Kinship in East London* have been influential in stressing the continuing importance of community in some parts of industrial society.[10] The theory of community care is implicitly based on an assumption that the community is alive and functioning, but what is the reality of community for most people in modern society? More specifically, to what extent does the community provide practical support to those people entrusted with the care of the severely mentally handicapped? Is the notion of community really relevant in this context?

Table 6.7: Participation of Relatives, Friends and Neighbours in Child Care and Housework

Task	Relatives = 334 100%		Friends = 147 100%		Neighbours = 107 100%	
	Partici-pant	Helper	Partici-pant	Helper	Partici-pant	Helper
Physical child care						
Dressing	0	5 (1.5%)	0	1 (0.7%)	0	0
Washing	0	1 (0.3%)	0	0	0	1 (0.9%)
Nappies	1 (0.3%)	0	0	0	0	1 (0.9%)
Toiletting	0	4 (1.2%)	0	0	0	1 (0.9%)
Feeding	0	4 (1.2%)	0	0	0	0
Lifting	0	4 (1.2%)	0	1 (0.7%)	0	1 (0.9%)
Child minding						
After school	2 (0.6%)	4 (1.2%)	0	1 (0.7%)	0	0
Weekends	3 (0.9%)	9 (2.7%)	2 (1.4%)	0	0	0
School holidays	4 (1.2%)	8 (2.5%)	0	3 (2.0%)	0	2 (1.9%)
Baby-sitting	2 (0.6%)	32 (9.6%)	0	7 (4.8%)	0	2. (1.9%)
Household tasks					0	
Cleaning	2 (0.6%)	2 (0.6%)	0	0	0	1 (0.9%)
Cooking	2 (0.6%)	2 (0.6%)	0	1 (0.7%)	0	0
Washing dishes	1 (0.3%)	6 (1.8%)	0	0	0	0
Washing clothes	1 (0.3%)	5 (1.5%)	0	0	0	0
Shopping	3 (0.9%)	8 (2.4%)	0	0	0	6 (5.6%)

Table 6.7 shows the extent of participation in chld care and housework of relatives, friends and neighbours of the families. In relation to the day-to-day practical burdens experienced by the mothers of these severely handicapped children, the impact of community was negligible for most. The earlier part of this chapter has commented on the relatively low level of participation by fathers and children in the domestic routine, but in comparison to others outside the nuclear family, their contribution was very high. The 588 relatives, friends and neighbours whom mothers saw at least once a month provided only 146 instances of help with the daily domestic routine, an average of 1.2 per family. Mothers may have received support in crises or emotional and psychological support from these people, but they certainly did not receive much help with the day-to-day practical burdens of providing care. The level of support provided by relatives, friends and neighbours was so low that there was little point in calculating the overall scores that were used to assess the contribution of fathers and siblings of the handicapped child.

Relatives

Both the mother's and her husband's relatives are included in Table 6.7. Mothers were asked which relatives they saw at least once a month, since it was assumed that those who were seen less frequently than this could not really be considered potential sources of support on a regular basis. Of those that mothers reported in this category, 85 per cent were the mother's own parents or siblings or her husband's parents or siblings. Nine relatives were living with the families, a further 117 lived within walking distance and a further 104 lived within the same town (i.e. a local bus ride away). Two-thirds were seen at least once a week and 56 per cent of these visited the respondent's own home. A comparison of these figures and the levels of support provided reveals the very small contribution they made to the families' daily routines. Large numbers of them were, at least potentially, available to provide support with the domestic routine, in the sense that they lived close enough and had regular contact with the families. In general, they were not involved in either child care or housework. More than three-quarters of the relatives regularly visited the mothers in their own homes. They were ideally placed to lend a hand with tasks such as keeping an eye on children for a while or helping with the shopping, but only twelve provided any help with minding children during the school holidays and only eleven regularly helped with the shopping. The task with which they provided most support was baby sitting, but this still only amounted to 10 per cent of the total number of relatives with whom families had regular contact.

Occasionally there were instances of relatives who provided an important, regular and reliable service. One mother had a sister living nearby who looked after her handicapped son every day after school:

> I get worn out chasing after Simon so I've got no patience left for the others. I work full time but if I didn't I'd run out of patience altogether. Being at work keeps me sane. My sister collects him from school and she keeps him till I get home, otherwise I couldn't work and I think he would have to go into care or something.

In this case, support with a specific task made the difference between being able to cope and having to give up the struggle. In other cases support from relatives was less frequent but no less valuable. One family relied on the husband's brother to take their handicapped daughter on holiday every summer with their family, but such help was the exception rather than the rule. Even more exceptional were the four families in which a relative provided daily support with various aspects of physical child care and housework, but in all of these the relative was living with the family. Although a number of studies have reported differences between the level of support provided by mother's and father's relatives these differences were not found in this study, where the level of support was uniformly low for both groups.

The point was made earlier in this chapter that the fact that most fathers made only minimal contributions to the domestic routine was largely accepted by their wives. The same was true of relatives' contributions. Mothers did not expect much in the way of help from their relatives and the relatives in turn did not offer much. The relationship between the nuclear family and its kinship network in modern socieites was discussed at some length in Chapter 3, where it was pointed out that, in spite of evidence that kinship networks have continued to be important in certain respects, their role as providers of day-to-day support with the domestic routine has become increasingly irrelevant to the needs of most families in a relatively affluent society which also has the provisions of a welfare state. The long-term dependence of one family member means that such support would be of great value to the family with a handicapped child, but patterns of support reflect the needs of the majority of families rather than the special needs of those faced with particular problems. Thus it was not surprising that these families received relatively little in the way of practical help from their relatives.

Whilst the very small contribution relatives made to the domestic routine has been justifiably stressed, it should be stated that most mothers nevertheless valued the social contact they had with kin and the feeling that they could, if necessary, call on them in time of crisis. Relatives tended to be more accepting of the handicapped child's behaviour than did other people. Since many families found their social lives outside the home severely curtailed, mutual visiting of kin was the their only opportunity to spend time with other people. However, some families found that even relatives were not prepared to accept a handicapped child:

We don't see a lot of my sister-in-law and her family since Karen was born. She told my husband that she felt uncomfortable with Karen. She came round a couple of times but she didn't even look at Karen. If people can't accept her as she is, then I would rather they didn't come round.

There is another element in the relationship between the family and the kinship network which has so far not been mentioned. Like children, relatives can provide support but they can also place additional demands on the family's resources, and particularly on the mother's resources. It is difficult to assess the importance of this but it can be a major factor in individual situations. In some cases an elderly parent lived with the family, thus bringing another dependent person into the household, and in others the mother had to visit parents regularly and help them with the housework, shopping, etc. The difficulties faced by Sheila's mother were described in the previous chapter but, in addition to these, she also had to devote time to her own and her husband's father. The latter only required visiting regularly, but she also had to wash and to do the shopping for her own father. The increasing dependency of relatives as they grow older tends to occur at a time when the mother herself is older and therefore finds things more difficult to cope with, when problems presented by the handicapped child are often becoming worse and when older children are beginning to leave home, therefore reducing the amount of support that they can provide. In a society in which the numbers of very old and therefore very dependent people are increasing rapidly, this problem is likely to affect more families with a handicapped child.

Friends and Neighbours

The problem of social isolation which many parents of handicapped children face has already been mentioned on a number of occasions. The mothers mentioned a total of 147 friends whom they saw at least once a month, but almost 40 per cent of mothers said they had nobody whom they would classify as a friend. The handicapped child often severely restricted the opportunity to make friends, but in addition, some mothers found that they had actually lost friends since the birth of the handicapped child. They found that the child's behaviour presented insurmountable problems which meant that it was easier not to maintain friendships:

> I would like to be able to visit friends and for my friends to visit me. Most people get embarrassed when she [the handicapped child] is there and she makes a mess everywhere. I would be upset myself. They would probably understand but I am over-sensitive. I would just like to live a normal life.

However, it should be borne in mind that the lack of friendships

among these mothers was not solely a consequence of having a handicapped child, but also of their socially isolated position as housewives.
The child was often indirectly responsible for the fact that they were
tied to the home, but many mothers of normal children also face
similar problems of social isolation. It is clear from Table 6.7 that
friends were in a different category from relatives when it came to the
provision of practical support. There were only three instances of help
from friends with physical child care and household tasks and only
thirteen with child minding. In the two instances where friends shared
the minding of children at weekends this was a reciprocal relationship
in which the respondents also minded their friends' children. In general
though, there seemed to be no obligation upon friends to help out in a
practical way and, whilst relatives were often expected to be available
to help deal with crises, this did not seem to be expected of friends.

The idea of the neighbourhood support network which helps those
in need has played a large part in the arguments advanced by the
advocates of community care. The idea owes much to literary and
sociological writings on traditional working-class communities. The
mothers in this study were asked if they had any neighbours of whom
they could ask a favour or from whom they could borrow things. This
was essentially a hypothetical category in that it did not necessarily
indicate that the mother actually utilised these services on a day-to-day
basis. Even so, only 107 neighbours were reported in this category by
the mothers and exactly half reported that they knew nobody in this
category. In other words there was nobody in the neighbourhood on
whom they felt they could call if they needed help. This hardly seems
to constitute care by the community. For those mothers who did have
a neighbour on whom they could call, this was usually only a hypothetical source of support. It is clear from Table 6.7 that the help
actually provided by neighbours did not constitute a major contribution
to the daily routine. There were only 15 instances of any help with the
domestic routine on a regular basis from neighbours. However, just as
social contact and support in crises was valued when it was available
from relatives it was also important when provided by neighbours.
Heather's mother received no regular practical support from her neighbours but she said: 'The people in the neighbourhood can be relied
upon for help when necessary. We pop in and out of each others houses
for coffee.'

Discussion

In terms of support inside and outside the family the results obtained in this study apparently contradict the findings of most other similar studies. Hewitt described half of the fathers in her study as highly participant in the domestic routine and Bayley reported that 40 per cent of fathers contributed much help.[11] In contrast, only a quarter of fathers in this study contributed a high level of support and it was pointed out that even this level was not very high when compared with the amount of work necessary. There is little reference in other studies to the role played by siblings of the handicapped child, thus comparisons between this and other studies in this respect are not possible. With respect to extra familial support Jaehnig reported that 60 per cent of families were receiving some help from neighbours.[12] Bayley reported that 70 per cent of families received considerable support from neighbours and Carr that half of the families she studied had a good deal of support from relatives.[13] In the whole of this study there were 146 instances of help with the daily routine from relatives and 15 instances of help from neighbours.

Why should there be such a discrepancy between this study and those mentioned above? There is no evidence that families in this study were different from those in other studies in terms of their composition, social class, area of residence, etc. The reasons for the large discrepancy lie in the sorts of tasks studied and the ways in which levels of support were defined. Thus help with such things as money, decorating and gardening was not included and no allowance was made for people who might be called upon in times of special need. However, this alone could not account for the reported differences. The principal reason for the lack of agreement between this and other studies appears to be the way in which different levels of support were defined. None of the studies referred to above systematically collected information about what individuals actually did with respect to a wide range of domestic tasks. Terms such as 'frequent', 'considerable support', 'a good deal', and 'highly participant' imply relative standards and these are never expliticitly defined in the studies referred to. It appears that they are relative to the level achieved by other fathers, other relatives or other neighbours, but there is no reference to the overall amount of work necessary or to the amount that the mothers did. There is no way of knowing whether, for example, the overall level of support provided by fathers was low, since the standard was only relative to other fathers. It is interesting that Hewett in her study of families with a cerebral palsied child, reported that fathers' level of participation was similar to that observed in normal families.[14] One of the only systematic studies of what fathers actually do in normal families reported that 60 per cent had a low level of participation.[15] This compares with the 52 per cent found in this study and is probably a more realistic estimate of the realities of the daily domestic routine for most mothers.

In conclusion, it can be said that, in reality, the term community care for a mentally handicapped child refers to care *in* the community but not care *by* the community. The nuclear family is the framework in which the child is cared for. Within the family it is mothers who carry the major burden of care usually with relatively little support from other family members. The contribution of people outside the family to the practical burden of care is almost negligible.

7 THE SERVICES

The historical development of services for the mentally handicapped and their families was briefly reviewed in Chapter 1 of this book. Although services for this group have been a Cinderella among the wider provisions of the developing welfare state throughout the last century, there have been improvements in education, health and social services provisions, partly as a consequence of the desire to seek alternatives to institutional care for the mentally handicapped. However, it was pointed out in Chapter 1 that advocating community care was not necessarily the same thing as actually providing the services that would affect the day-to-day lives of the mentally handicapped and their families. Have we really seen the flowering of what Titmuss described in 1961 as the everlasting cottage garden trailer – community care?[1] Notable improvements include better educational provisions, financial support through the Constant Attendance Allowance and, more recently, the Mobility Allowance, practical support through the Rowntree Trust and the provision of more and better residential accommodation. But it is important to assess just how much these developments have affected the day-to-day lives of the majority of families with a handicapped member. Also we must be aware of the changing needs of families and seek to determine the ways in which services require further developments.

A detailed evaluation of the full range of services provided for the mentally handicapped and their families was not a central objective of the study described here. The main emphasis was on the organisation of the day-to-day domestic routine which constitutes the essence of community care, but sufficient information was collected to allow a broad assessment of the contribution made by services and how this affected the day-to-day lives of the families. This information is presented in this chapter and, although detailed prescriptions for improvements in the current services are left until the final chapter, the problems that families experienced and some of the ways in which these might have been overcome are discussed. An important objective was to compare the levels of services received by the home and admissions groups, in order to establish to what extent the decision to seek long-term institutional care for the handicapped child was related to the support available from the services. Therefore, tables which compare

147

the home and admissions groups in terms of services received include only those families which were matched on the basis of the handicapped child's age and social quotient. Thus differences shown in the levels of services received by the two groups were not a reflection of grossly different problems in the management of the handicapped child. However, although the home and admissions groups were broadly comparable in terms of the handicapped children, some allowance has to be made for the fact that they were drawn from different geographical areas. The level and quality of education, health and social services varies considerably from one area another. Therefore, in this discussion of services, note is made of geographical variations which may explain some of the differences between the two groups. The services are dealt with under five headings: education, health, social services, voluntary services and short-term care. Short-term care is dealt with separately because of its importance to families and because it was provided by a number of different agencies.

Education

The transfer of responsibility for education from health to education authorities, achieved in the same year as the production of the White Paper, *Better Services for the Mentally Handicapped*, has led to considerable improvements in the education of the mentally handicapped. The number of places available in special schools has increased considerably, although there remain areas in which the level of provision is still unsatisfactory. In particular, there are many more places available in special care classes for profoundly handicapped children. However, the quality of education is much more difficult to assess and controversy continues over the question of whether it is desirable to provide education in special schools or whether mentally handicapped children should be taught in ordinary schools. The recent report of the Warnock Committee, which will probably form the basis of future policy, came out in favour of the continuing use of special schools but recommended many improvements, including increased contact and collaboration with ordinary schools.[2] Educational provision for the children in this study was quite good. All of the schools had special care units to cater for the most severely handicapped children and no child was excluded from school. The physical facilities and staffing ratios in most schools were at least as good as the national average. Most of the schools also had the services of a physiotherapist for the physically handicapped children for at least a short time each week, but there was marked lack of other specialists such as speech therapists.

In spite of the various deficiencies in the educational system that mothers mentioned it was, of all the services, the one that had most impact on the families' daily routines. Its contribution was two-fold in that the child's attendance at school both relieved the mothers of the burden of care and helped the child to develop skills which would ultimately reduce that burden through his or her increasing independence. The first contribution was very important to virtually all the mothers. For many of them, the time that the handicapped child spent at school was the only time during which they could feel free of their caring responsibilities, since even when other family members were around they could not be relied upon to take full responsibility for the child. The significance of the second type of contribution depended very much on the child's level of development and therefore the rate at which he or she could be expected to learn. For mothers of the most profoundly handicapped children, development was often non-existent or so slow as to be almost imperceptible. Mothers of more able children on the other hand, noticed real developments, such as learning to dress or learning to go to the toilet alone, which they attributed to the school's influence and which also had a great impact on the ordinary domestic routine.

Table 7.1: Education Day Care

Education/day care	Home	Admissions	Total
None	1 (3%)	1 (3%)	2 (3%)
School hours	29 (97%)	27 (90%)	56 (93%)
More than school hours	0	2 (7%)	2 (3%)
Total (100%)	30	30	60

Table 7.1 shows the number of children in the matched groups who were receiving education or day care. Only two children were not attending school or some form of day centre, although these had not been excluded from school. Both were under five years of age and, although all areas included in the study provided facilities at school for children of three years of age, these parents did not wish to send their child to school until he or she reached the age of five. Other studies in other areas have reported that some handicapped children were excluded because schools did not have sufficient facilities to cope with them.[3] Although there may still be

some areas in which families are unable to obtain appropriate education for their handicapped child, it is likely that such problems are much less common than they were 20 or even 10 years ago. As mentioned above, all of the schools had special care units capable of caring for the most profoundly handicapped children, although there were sometimes problems in accommodating children with severe behaviour problems. Only one child had, however, been excluded because of behaviour problems, and this was a number of years prior to the study. The school had felt unable to cope with the problems this twelve-year-old boy presented, but the family managed to find alternative accommodation at a day centre attached to a residential unit. Two children, both in the admissions group, who presented behavioural problems were receiving day care for periods longer than normal school hours and were also able to receive care during part of the school holidays. These two were also attending day centres attached to residential units.

Mothers were not asked to comment directly upon any of the services, but, in the course of the interview, many mothers offered comments and these were recorded. Although there were no problems in obtaining day care for the handicapped child, this should not be taken to imply that the provisions were considered satisfactory in all respects by all mothers. The majority, however, praised the work that the teachers did in helping their child to develop. The following comment was characteristic of many:

> Her teacher at the moment is marvellous. She is full of ideas and seems to keep the children constantly occupied and helps them . . . She is the one that I find easiest to talk to. They always seem to welcome visitors and they are happy to discuss any problems.

Comments which expressed dissatisfaction with the child's performance at school and therefore with the way in which he or she was being taught were rare, although it is difficult to know whether mothers who made no comment were critical of these things. Mrs Evans complained that Gary had not made any progress at school:

> There's a girl across the road comes in during the school holidays. He seems to improve more talking to her than he does at school. He has just got cheeky since he's gone to school. He just copies the other kids. He is stuck with a load of mongolians but he's not like them.

Apart from the criticisms of the education that their child was receiving, many mothers complained that school hours were too short. As many as 31 per cent wanted their children to attend school for longer hours and 68 per cent wanted more help during the school holidays. These and other perceived needs for additional support will be dealt with in more detail in the following chapter. There were, however, a number of other problems that mothers raised in relation to educational facilities. The main category of critical comments was that relating to problems of getting the children to and from school. The severely physically handicapped children were collected from their homes by an ambulance service and returned in the afternoon, whilst most of the remainder travelled on the school bus service. There were few complaints about the ambulance service since it called at the child's home, although the timing was sometimes unreliable. Many of the parents whose children went on the bus, however, were very critical. The children had to be taken to a collection point where they sometimes had to wait for half an hour or longer, and returning in the afternoon to meet them from the bus often involved a similar wait. Some children were not scheduled to be collected by the bus service until 9.30 a.m. and they were returned at 3.30 p.m. This meant that the time during which mothers were effectively relieved of the responsibility of caring for the child was very short, and apart from the discomfort and inconvenience of waiting on the street, the fact that the bus could not be relied upon to be on time made it very difficult for mothers to commit themselves to activities at particular times. For some, the possibility of even part-time employment was ruled out because they could not guarantee to arrive on time:

> You never know when the bus is going to come, once last winter it didn't arrive at all. Sometimes we have to wait for half an hour or more. It's alright at this time of year [summer] but its not much fun in the winter. I had a job in the supermarket last year but I had to give it up because I kept coming in late and the manager didn't like it.

Another problem which, like bussing, was also related to the distance between home and school, was the difficulty of maintaining contact with the teachers. Most parents could not see the teacher when taking their child to school or collecting them as they might have done with their normal children because they usually lived some miles away from the school and were forced to use the school bus service. This meant

that the only opportunity many of them had to meet and discuss the
child's progress with the teacher was at the relatively infrequent
parents' evenings at school. Some parents found that even this was
impossible because of the difficulty of finding a suitable baby-sitter.
For some the only information available was from the supervisor on the
school bus. This sometimes meant that when their child came home
with a cut or bruise they were unable to find out what happened and
mothers found this both worrying and annoying. Those parents who did
feel that they had sufficient contact with the teachers were the ones
who either took their children to school themselves because they
happened to live close by or were able to take them by car, and those
who were able to maintain telephone contact with the school. Some of
the mothers who had attended parents' evenings felt that there was
insufficient opportunity to discuss things in detail. A number offered
constructive suggestions such as Mrs Stanley:

> I don't think there's enough time for individual parents at these
> meetings. I think it would be best if they invited you individually to
> see the teachers or something like that. You could probably go for
> an hour or so on your own to see the teacher.

Many of the mothers' criticisms of the schools raised, often indirectly,
the question of whether or not mentally handicapped children should
be segregated from other children for educational purposes. The debate
on this issue has tended to be conducted around the educational and
social needs of the handicapped child, but it is important to take
account of the parents' feelings about the situation and to recognise
that, in addition to meeting the children's needs, the schools also provide much needed relief for mothers. Mothers in this study were not
asked how they felt about whether their child should be educated in a
special school, but a number volunteered the information that they
would prefer him or her to go to local schools. In some cases this was
for purely practical reasons and in others because they felt that he or
she would make more progress at an ordinary school. In addition, two
mothers said that their child should go to the local school because they
felt that it was important that other children in the area learned to
accept and understand handicapped children. This may, in the long run,
be one of the strongest arguments in favour of integration. In its
broadest sense the education of the rest of society is fundamental to an
improvement in conditions for the mentally handicapped and their
families. Nevertheless, the special schools have much to offer the

mentally handicapped child which it may not be possible to provide in normal schools, and the majority of mothers interviewed held the schools in very high esteem.

The Health Services

The role of the health services in the care of the mentally handicapped has undergone many changes in the past 50 years. The emphasis has shifted from a concentration on ascertainment and custodial care to assessment, treatment and community care. Responsiblity for education has passed to the education authority and social services departments have begun to play a much bigger role in the provision of community support and residential care for the less severely handicapped. These developments do not, however, seem to have resulted in a clarification of the roles of the various health service professions in the care and treatment of the mentally handicapped. General practitioners, district nurses, community mental handicap nurses, health visitors, community physicians, paediatricians, hospital nurses, mental handicap specialists and a range of other medical specialists are involved in varying degrees, but their roles seem to depend largely on individual interest and local circumstances. One of the reasons for this variability and confusion is the often inadequate attention given to this group in the training of the various professions. The children often require specialist assessment and treatment for their mental and physical handicaps but they and their families also require treatment, care and advice from a range of non-specialists. Thus it is essential that these people have sufficient knowledge to be able to provide treatment, care and advice which is appropriate to the circumstances. The experiences of families with the health services reflect this variability and confusion, some reporting mainly positive experiences and others mostly negative.

Table 7.2 shows the level of contact that families in the matched home and admissions groups had with the health services in terms of the number having had recent contact with each of the services. In all cases more children in the home group had recent contact than those in the admissions group. It is probable that this reflected a different emphasis in the different areas on the care of the mentally handicapped as a health service responsibility. In Salford, where families in the home group lived, there was a long tradition of health service involvement in the care of mentally handicapped, both in the hospital services and in the community health services. This probably goes a long way towards explaining the higher level of contact that children from the home group had with the health services.

Table 7.2: The Health Services

	Home N = 30 (100%)	Admissions N = 30 (100%)	Total N = 60 (100%)
General practitioner			
Seen GP in last 3 months	21 (70%)	15 (50%)	36 (60%)
Seen GP in last year	5 (17%)	9 (30%)	14 (23%)
1 year since last contact with GP	4 (13%)	6 (20%)	10 (17%)
District nurse/HV			
Seen DN or HV in past year	8 (27%)	2 (7%)	10 (17%)
Not seen DN or HV in past year	22 (73%)	28 (93%)	50 (83%)
School doctor			
Seen school doctor in past year	27 (90%)	20 (67%)	47 (78%)
Not seen school doctor in past year	3 (10%)	10 (33%)	13 (22%)
Hospital doctor			
Seen hospital doctor in past year	19 (63%)	16 (53%)	35 (58%)
Not seen hospital doctor in past year	11 (37%)	14 (47%)	25 (42%)

Of the children in the home group, 70 per cent had seen their GP in the three months preceding the interview, compared with only 50 per cent of those in the admissions group. The majority of consultations with GPs were for minor physical ailments and there is no reason to suppose that the Salford children experienced more of these than children in the other areas, but it is likely that consultation rates for such problems were affected by expectations about whether or not the GP would be sympathetic and helpful. The attention devoted to the problems of the mentally handicapped in Salford by hospital and community services may also have influenced the knowledge and attitudes of general practitioners. By and large mothers did not expect a great deal from their GPs. They wanted advice and information about the nature of the child's condition and prospects for the future, particularly during the early years, and they wanted treatment for the usual range of childhood illnesses which took account of the special circumstances of a family with a mentally handicapped child. Some GPs were unwilling to spare the time to offer advice and information but the majority were unable to provide these things because they were largely ignorant of the condition. In treating straightforward physical illnesses,

GPs often failed to take into account the difficulty some mothers had in persuading the child to complete the prescribed course of treatment. In other cases doctors refused to accept as worthy of medical intervention, problems in the handicapped child which affected the mother's own health. Philip's mother might have found things a lot easier if her general practitioner had viewed her problems sympathetically at an earlier stage:

> The problem was the first five years when he didn't sleep. I didn't sleep because of him and I couldn't build my strength up to cope with him. I used to tell the doctor I only got half an hours' sleep but he just didn't believe me. In the end the clinic welfare worker went to my doctor because she saw I was at the end of my tether. I feel 10 years older than I am.

Contact with community nursing services was extremely low, only 17 per cent of families having seen a district nurse or health visitor during the previous year. Eight of the ten children who had been seen were in the home group, although two of these had only been seen incidentally whilst the nurse was visiting another family member. All of the children for whom specific visits had been made were under seven years of age and it is likely that most of these contacts were continuations of contacts which had started shortly after birth. The frequency of visiting seemed to decline as the child grew older and, in the majority of cases, it ceased soon after he or she reached school age, unless a specific visit was requested. Such specific visits were usually for the provision of disposable nappies or rubber sheets for incontinent children, but some mothers reported that they were a waste of time since they still had to attend the welfare clinic in order to obtain a regular supply of disposable nappies. At the time the study was conducted there were no specialist community mental handicap nurses working in the area. Such specialists are still few and far between, but the fact that attention is being devoted to the special needs of the mentally handicapped and their families for a community nursing service holds out the hope for improvements in the future.

Most severely mentally handicapped children undergo a routine medical check-up at school approximately once a year. It was reported that 78 per cent of children had been seen by the school medical officer in the previous twelve months, but once again there was a higher proportion in the home group than the admissions group (90 per cent compared with 67 per cent). However, the accuracy of these figures is doubtful since some mothers may not even have been aware that the check-up had been carried out at school. It is possible that since the health services seemed to have more contact with home group families, these mothers were more likely to know that a check-up had been carried out at school. Whether or not such check-ups were useful to the parents very much depended upon the individual doctor. In some cases the check-up provided an opportunity to discuss the child's progress and problems, but in many instances mothers were either unable to attend the check-up or, when they did, found the doctor unwilling to listen to them or to answer questions.

Finally, 58 per cent of children had seen a hospital specialist of one sort or another during the previous year, the home group once again having a slightly higher level of contact than the admissions group. This higher level of contact was probably due to the physical proximity of specialist services and the keen interest shown by certain consultants. A large children's hospital is situated in Salford and a mental handicap hospital just outside the city. Information was collected on the type of hospital specialist seen and the reason for consultation. The largest category of consultations was for routine checks with paediatricians and mental handicap consultants. The children in the admissions group had more contact with the latter while those in the home group had more contact with the paediatricians. These checks were usually to assess the child's progress, review medical treatment and discuss any problems. Most of the consultations with mental handicap specialists took place while the child was in short-term care or as part of the procedure for allocating places for long-term hospital accommodation. Comments on mental handicap and paediatric specialists were generally favourable, although as with other doctors, some mothers complained of an un-willingness to discuss problems fully. Comments on other specialists were, on the whole less favourable, since the mothers felt that they were often unaware of the problems of caring for a mentally handi-capped child.

In general, the health services had little obvious direct impact on the problems of day-to-day care of the majority of handicapped children. Mothers' experiences of contact with doctors and nurses were extremely varied and their evaluation of the services offered was often dependent on the attitudes of the individuals with whom they had contact. Some doctors were highly praised for their sympathy, patience, understanding and willingness to spend time answering questions in a language the mothers could understand. On the other hand, some were criticised because they lacked these same characteristics. This was true of both

the community and hospital-based health service personnel. A
sympathetic doctor to whom they could turn for advice and help was a
great asset to many parents, but whether this was a GP, paediatrician,
mental handicap consultant, paediatric neurologist or any other
specialist did not seem to be of great importance. Graham's mother
referred to a paediatrician in this way, although she regretted that the
level of contact had declined as he became older:

> . . . if I had any problems I would always ring Dr Jones and he'd
> make an appointment for me to go over and see him. He had a full
> assessment every three months at first and then every six months. I
> used to enjoy going. I would have liked for it to have continued
> because if you go and have a child assessed like that you have a good
> idea how they are getting on.

Similarly, Stephen's mother always felt she could rely on her GP: 'Oh, I
call him out straight away. You know, for anything. I just call him and
he comes and puts things right for me. He is a good doctor. I would go
mad if anything ever happened to him.' These comments suggest that an
important part of the doctor's role in relation to the mentally handicapped is the provision of information, support and advice which may
be unrelated to his or her capacity to provide medical treatment. Those
parents who had not been able to develop such a relationship with a
doctor tended to express criticisms of the health services in general and
the doctors in particular, whereas those who had such a relationship
were more likely to be critical of specific aspects of the services, rather
than to generalise their criticisms. Many doctors were described by
parents as not knowing very much about mental handicap and not
seeming to care very much either. Mrs Gordon's comments were similar
to those of many other mothers:

> My own doctor doesn't seem to have any idea what it's like having a
> handicapped kiddy. I only go when she's got something wrong with
> her. The school doctor doesn't really understand Carol either. She
> had her check-up yesterday. When he got hold of her feet she kicked
> up towards his face, and when he tried to put her on the scales she
> jumped up and grabbed his tie, she nearly choked him. You can't
> talk to him. Not like Dr Smith at the hospital.

Social Services

Like education and health, social services for families with a mentally handicapped member have changed considerably in the past ten years as a result of the reorganisation of social services that followed the Seebohm Report in 1968. Whilst the old system, where mental welfare officers were responsible for the provision of social services for this group, had many deficiencies, the reorganisation has not greatly benefited most families with a mentally handicapped child. Work with this group forms only a small part of the total responsibilities of social services departments, and we have witnessed a steady decline in the numbers of specialist social workers with the knowledge and experience necessary to deal with the problems of such groups as the severely mentally handicapped. The emphasis on genericism in social work has meant that the training and experience of social workers necessarily concentrates on the needs of the largest groups, such as the elderly and the mentally ill, often to the exclusion of smaller groups. At the same time as reorganisation has created problems in the provision of support services for families with a mentally handicapped member, two other factors have resulted in increasing the pressure on these services. First, recent years have seen a sharp increase in the demand for social services from other groups, particularly the elderly; and secondly, cash limits have been imposed on the resources available to meet the problems. The curtailment of public expenditure in order to deal with economic problems has affected the work of many social services departments, the worst affected area being community support services. In the light of these developments it was not surprising that the support provided to families in this study often left a lot to be desired.

Table 7.3: Social Services

	Home N = 30 (100%)	Admissions N = 30 (100%)	Total N = 60 (100%)
Social worker			
Seen social worker in past 3 months	12 (40%)	19 (63%)	31 (52%)
Seen social worker in past year	5 (17%)	6 (20%)	11 (18%)
Not seen social worker in past year	13 (43%)	5 (17%)	18 (30%)
Other social services			
Yes	2 (7%)	12 (40%)	14 (23%)
No	28 (93%)	18 (60%)	46 (77%)

It was noted in the previous section that families in the home group had considerably more contact with various health service personnel than did those in the admissions group, but this situation was sharply reversed in respect of social services. Admissions group families had both a higher level of contact with social workers and received more additional services. It was, of course, to be expected that the families of children referred to the study by social workers would report a higher level of contact with social workers, and all of these families had been visited by a social worker during the previous year. However, families of children whose name was on a hospital waiting list also had a much higher level of contact with social workers than did the home group. As many as 83 per cent of admissions group families had seen a social worker in the previous year compared with only 57 per cent of those in the home group, yet even annual contact represented a very minimal commitment on the part of the social services departments. Of all the families, almost half had not seen a social worker in the previous three months, and thus could hardly be described as being in regular contact with their social worker.

Mothers were asked whether they had received any other services from the social services department. These included a laundry service, special transport, providing a telephone and arranging for alterations to housing. Only 23 per cent of families had received any direct service of this nature, although many more would have benefited from the provision of such services. Many parents did not possess the knowledge and skills which often seemed to be necessary to obtain direct support. Unless the social worker took it upon her/himself to obtain services, parents had to know what services they were entitled to, who to approach, how to present their case and, above all, to be prepared for a long and arduous struggle with bureaucracy. It was not surprising therefore, that many families either did not know what services they were entitled to or, if they did, had given up the struggle to obtain them. Families who were fortunate enough to have received services tended to be those who had regular contact with a social worker. Thus 40 per cent of admissions group families, who had more contact with social workers, had received services compared with only 7 per cent of those in the home group.

Criticisms of the social workers and social services departments were very common, even among those families who had been visited and had received additional services. Many mothers complained that visits by social workers simply wasted time that they could have spent doing other things. They said that the social workers knew very little about the problems of caring for a mentally handicapped child. Some felt that the visits were of more use to the social worker than they were to themselves, since at least the social worker learned a little about mental handicap. Very few found a short chat over a cup of tea useful, since on the one hand no practical help was offered, and on the other hand there was insufficient time to discuss problems with somebody who had very little understanding of the situations faced by families. The following quote from one of the mothers illustrates the ambiguity of the relationship between social worker and parent:

> I don't think they're much use really, the ones I've come across anyway. One came a couple of weeks back, I don't know what she came for. She just came in and sat down, 'I'm Mrs Martin'. Not much use at all really. She just asked the children's names. I said, 'This one is Graham'. Well that was it. She said goodbye then. I don't know what they come for really.

There were some mothers however, particularly among the admissions group, who spoke highly of their social workers and had managed to develop a relationship which provided necessary services and someone to talk to who could understand their problems. Others said that they had had this sort of relationship in the past when they had been visited by the mental welfare officer, but that in recent years they had been visited by a succession of social workers who seemed to have no specialised knowledge.

What many families wanted from the social services departments was not a chat over a cup of tea, but practical support that met their particular needs. The availability of such support varied from area to area, from social worker to social worker and from family to family. Whilst one family was able to obtain a grant for half the cost of building a special extension for a child who was severely physically handicapped, including bedroom, bathroom, toilet and an electric hoist between bedroom and bathroom, another was unable to persuade the social services department to provide a ramp for a wheel chair and to enlarge the doors inside the house to accommodate the wheel chair. Others had tried asking social workers for help with a wide range of problems, but usually with little success. A number of families lived in substandard housing and had attempted to enlist the social worker's help in getting re-housed. Mrs Marshall had had little success in this:

> There's nowhere for Michael to play. He hates coming home to this slum. Most of my problems would be helped if we could get a better

place to live. I can't let any of the children out to play. All the social worker says is 'We will see what can be done'. She has been saying that for a year now.

In other instances social workers either did not understand the problem or did not know where to obtain special equipment which would have eased the problem. Sarah presented a problem at night because she was very restless, frequently uncovered herself and occasionally fell out of bed. Her mother said:

She could do with a type of sleeping bag to fasten her in but I don't know if they are on the market. I'm up and down the stairs like a yo-yo. At the hospital they put her in a sort of waistcoat which allows them plenty of freedom, and it has strings at each side and they can fasten her into the bed so she can't get out. I'd be delighted to buy her one of these but I don't know where to get one from. I asked the social worker but she didn't know where to get them. She didn't seem to understand what I was on about.

Those families who did succeed in obtaining practical support often had to be extremely persistent. Mrs Watson commented:

If we want anything done we have to phone Social Services head office. Our own social worker never calls unless we ask her to. She says 'I'll ring you back', but she never does. This new social worker would be no use to people who were new to it all. She doesn't seem to know what to do herself.

Finally, there were services which might, in theory, have been available, but which mothers either did not think of asking for or felt that it was a waste of time to ask. The heavy burden of housework that many mothers experienced was stressed in earlier chapters, but none of the mothers in the study was receiving or had ever received the services of a home help, and although 42 per cent of the children were frequently incontinent only one mother had ever been offered a laundry service. The provision of this sort of practical support on a day-to-day basis would have made an enormous difference to some families.

The overall low level of support provided by social services departments and the concentration of what support was available among those whose child was awaiting admission to long-term care, reflects a service oriented to crisis rather than to continuing long-term support. The mere fact of having a severely mentally handicapped child was insufficient to warrant regular contact with a social worker and the provision of specialised support services. It seemed that only when additional problems were identified, such as a demand for long-term residential care, did a particular family situation become a legitimate area of concern for the social worker. Some social services departments had a policy of maintaining contact with all families with a mentally handicapped member, but this was becoming more and more a formality as services came under increasing pressure. Some had, in the past, been visited regularly but this had declined in recent years. In order for social services support to be effective, social workers must possess a knowledge of the general problems of mental handicap, the services available and also the specific circumstances of individual families. Only in this way is it possible to anticipate needs and meet them with practical support which is relevant to the family's day-to-day domestic routine. It was a telling comment on the present state of services that many mothers commented, at the end of the research interview, that the two hours they had spent talking to the interviewer had been of much greater value than had the visits they received from a social worker. One of the mothers telephoned the author two years after the original interview to ask for advice. She said: 'You were the only person I could think to ask for help.'

Voluntary Services

Voluntary agencies continue to play a very important part in increasing public awareness of the problems of mental handicap, campaigning for better services, providing information on services available and actually giving practical help to families. The fact that these organisations are independent of the various statutory services gives them a certain advantage in meeting the needs of particular groups such as the mentally handicapped, and also means that families are sometimes prepared to seek their help when they do not wish to approach statutory services or have been turned away by these agencies. The government has increasingly recognised the importance of voluntary organisations and is attempting to channel financial support to them to help them provide services. One of the most important developments in this direction was the £3,000,000 fund for congenitally handicapped children set up by the government in 1973. This fund was given to the Joseph Rowntree Memorial Trust to administer, providing financial assistance to families usually for the purchase of household equipment. The other main organisation providing practical help for families is the National Society

for Mentally Handicapped Children, whose services include social work,
residential care and holidays. In addition to these, local charities and
parents groups often provide parties, outings, play schemes, etc. for
handicapped children. Such voluntary support should receive further
encouragement but, whilst the government's intention of providing
more assistance to voluntary bodies must be welcomed, it is important
that such developments should not be seen as alternatives to the provision of better statutory services.

Table 7.4: Voluntary Services

Have you received any voluntary services?	Home	Admissions	Total
Yes	5 (17%)	14 (47%)	19 (32%)
No	25 (83%)	16 (53%)	41 (68%)
Total (100%)	30	30	60

Voluntary organisations contributed a sizeable proportion of the
practical support available to the families in this study. Table 7.4 shows
the proportion of families who had received some sort of aid from
voluntary agencies. In fact, more families (32 per cent) had received
help from a voluntary service than had been aided in practical ways by
social services departments (23 per cent). However, more than half the
families who had received help from a voluntary agency had received
this from the Joseph Rowntree Trust. These grants were usually to
enable the family to buy a washing machine or drier and, in one case, to
assist in the purchase of a car. Services provided by other voluntary
agencies, usually locally based, included outings and parties and, in one
area, the opening of a special school for two weeks during the summer
holidays, staffed by volunteers. This sort of co-operative venture
between voluntary and statutory agencies may offer the possibility of
considerable improvements in services, although unfortunately such
schemes are at present rare. In common with support provided by social
services departments, the distribution of help from voluntary agencies
was weighted in favour of those families whose child was awaiting
admission to long-term care. This suggests that there is a tendency, even
on the part of the voluntary agencies, to concentrate their activities on
families who feel they can no longer cope with the problems, although
the higher level of contact that admissions group families had with
social workers must have been partly responsible for the fact that they
received more voluntary services, since it was often the social workers

who put them in touch with the voluntary agencies, particularly in the case of grants from the Rowntree Trust.

Short-term Care

Short-term residential care is provided for handicapped children in a wide variety of institutions by a number of different agencies. It is dealt with as a separate category here because of its importance as a practical service to families. The desirability of making short-term care facilities available to families has been stressed in numerous official publications, but there remains a grave shortage of suitable facilities in many areas. In addition to the shortage of places, historical development of institutional services for the mentally handicapped has meant that many of the available places are in large mental handicap hospitals which are often unsuited to providing this sort of care. More local residential units have been built in recent years which generally provide much better facilities, but many authorities have had difficulty in retaining a sufficient number of places for the provision of short-term accommodation. Voluntary organisations and private residential homes have done something to alleviate the problem, but there remains insufficient suitable accommodation to provide families with a respite from the strain of caring for their handicapped child. One imaginative alternative to institutional care is to make use of regular foster parents. A family is able to make its own arrangements with the foster parents and is provided with a certain number of credits to use in the course of a year. Such alternative solutions to the problem may be necessary in order to provide a sufficient level of provision, since the demand for short-term care tends to be concentrated at particular times of the year.

Table 7.5: Short-term Residential Care

Length of stay	Home	Social worker referrals	Total
None	18 (60%)	4 (13%)	22 (37%)
2 weeks	12 (40%)	6 (20%)	18 (30%)
2 – 4 weeks	0	8 (27%)	8 (13%)
4 weeks	0	12 (40%)	12 (20%)
Total (100%)	30	30	60

The short-term residential care received by children in this study was provided by the health service, social services, voluntary agencies and schools. All short-term care, irrespective of agency, is included in

Table 7.5 in order to provide an indication of the extent of this sort of support received by families. If day care at school is excluded, periods of short-term care were probably the most significant single item of support provided by the services, and the majority of children had received such care. Nevertheless, 37 per cent of all the children had received no short-term care in the twelve months preceding the interview, and a further 30 per cent had received less than two weeks. Some parents, particularly in the home group, were unaware of the availability of periods of short-term care, others had tried to find accommodation at a suitable time and failed and others had turned down offers of accommodation because of previous unpleasant experiences. Accommodation was provided in a large range of establishments, from large mental handicap hospitals to small homes run by voluntary agencies, but the bulk of accommodation was in the hospitals.

The discrepancy between the number of children in the home group who had received periods of short-term care and the number in the admissions group was even greater than the differences in contact with social workers. Only 40 per cent of home group children had had any short-term care in the previous year compared with 87 per cent of those awaiting admission, and 40 per cent of the latter had spent more than four weeks in short-term care. The limited availability of accommodation tends to result in its allocation on the basis of immediate need. If a long-term place could not be found, the next best thing was periods of short-term care. Thus families whose child was awaiting a long-term place were given priority in choosing the time when they wanted their child to be taken into short-term care, and efforts were made to provide accommodation for two weeks or more at a time. These families were also more likely to be in regular contact with the various agencies which provided short-term care. They tended to have regular contact with social workers and to attract the attention of voluntary organisations and, since they were already awaiting admission to long-term care, they were often in close contact with the same institutions that were capable of providing short-term care.

Those families who were receiving short-term care for their child sometimes expressed dissatisfaction with the accommodation provided and the way in which places were allocated. Most complaints about the nature of the accommodation and the care provided were directed at the mental handicap hospitals. Parents complained that their children lacked attention and stimulation and returned home in a poor state of health with behaviour problems they had not had before they left. However, an equal number of mothers praised the work of staff in these hospitals. It is impossible to say to what extent problems were caused by conditions in the hospital and to what extent they merely reflected the children's resistance to being sent away from home. Small group homes were sometimes criticised for the same reasons as the hospitals and in one case a mother found that a small home was unable to cope with her child:

> He was in short-term care for a while but he had a bad fit. Matron called an ambulance and sent him to hospital. The hospital said he was alright but the Matron sent him home. She said that they only had two night staff and wouldn't have him back in case he was bad again in the night. How would they have gone on if he'd been in permanent residential care and they couldn't have sent him back to us?

On the whole, the most satisfactory arrangements were those in which small residential units were available within easy reach of the family's own home, but these were very rare. Another family had looked high and low for suitable accommodation for their child.

> *They asked us* at the hospital *did we know* of places that were available! We went to Aberdeen, Bristol, St Albans, Stroud, Sussex and East Grinstead looking for places. There's a tremendous lack of communication and knowledge throughout the entire country.

The other main area of criticism was the way in which places were allocated. Some parents felt that the system was very unfair. They were unable to obtain suitable accommodation for their own child for two weeks but knew of others who had obtained up to six weeks accommodation at prime periods such as the summer holidays. Knowing the right people appeared to make a great difference to the availability of satisfactory short-term care. Some parents had developed contacts with staff in the hospitals and were able to telephone and reserve a place, others relied on social workers, others made requests through doctors and the remainder did not know whom to ask. Mrs Harris had found the social services department ineffecutual, but had found that her doctor achieved more success:

> I've had to ask and beg to get her a place. In fact when I ask Mrs Evans [social worker] she always says 'Oh all the places are full.' There's never any room. But when I ask my own doctor, and tell him

how ill I feel, he manages to get her away without any trouble. I've complained about this to the social services but they always say 'Oh Mrs Evans is very busy. She does other social work with old people.' The other social worker used to be much better at getting Susan a place in hospital.

In general, the parents who were most successful in obtaining accommodation when it was needed were those who were able to negotiate directly with the institutions they wanted their child to go to. Intermediaries such as social workers tended to make the process more difficult. Success in finding accommodation seemed to depend on whether the parents or the social worker had the necessary contacts with the people who controlled the availability of places.

Conclusions

With respect to the impact of services on the day-to-day lives of the majority of families with a severely mentally handicapped child, the findings of this study broadly parallel those of other research workers. Although services have undoubtedly improved over the years, there are not many areas in which this has had a great impact on the day-to-day problems faced by families. Tizard and Grad's study was conducted over 20 years ago, but in many respects their comments on the services are still applicable. Parents complained of doctors who lacked under-standing of their problems and whom they felt unable to ask important questions. They complained about educational facilities and about social workers who seemed to be of little help.[4] However, services did seem to have improved in two respects. First, Tizard and Grad reported that 83 per cent of pre-school children had no day care and 12 per cent of school-age children were excluded from school. Secondly, at the time their study was carried out, short-term care was only just becoming available and none of the families had benefited from this.[5] In both these respects the children in the present study were much better catered for, but on the other hand, the statutory requirement for supervision that existed in the 1950s meant that all families had regular contact with a specialist social worker. Tizard and Grad described this as: 'perhaps the most valuable social service available to the families . . .'.[6] This could hardly be said of the social work received by families in this study. In the past ten years other studies of the mentally handicapped and their families have made similar observations about the nature of services.[7] It is depressing to find that most families continue to lack much needed practical support and that most of the support provided is oriented towards crisis intervention rather than long-term preventive support.

Apart from the need for more resources to build more effective services for the mentally handicapped and their families, there are a number of problems within the present structure of services which inhibit their improvement. Four major problems came up time and again in the interviews.

1. Services are oriented to immediate crisis rather than long term prevention.

2. Professional roles are often ill-defined and not understood by either professional or client.

3. In some services there is a lack of *specialised* professionals with the requisite knowledge and understanding to deal with the problems.

4. There is often a marked lack of co-ordination between services and between different sections of the same service.

8 FELT NEEDS

That mothers of mentally handicapped children have many needs which are not being met, either by family, friends and relatives or by the statutory services, has already been implied in previous chapters. However, insufficient attention has so far been devoted to a systematic appraisal of the mothers' 'subjective' experience of needs. In so far as needs have been implied in earlier chapters, this has mostly been in terms of 'objective' criteria, although the quantitative data from the interviews has been supplemented with many quotes from mothers which illustrate now they felt about the problems. Since it is the mothers who, in most families, undertake the day-to-day care of the handicapped child, what they perceive as problematic and the extent to which they feel the need for additional support is of paramount importance in planning effective community support services. In this chapter, therefore, the mothers will be characterised in terms of their felt needs for additional support with the various aspects of the domestic routine.

The definition and measurement of needs is fundamental to the provision of adequate health and social services. Various ways of defining and measuring needs were discussed in Chapter 3, where it was pointed out that the choice of approach depends on the nature of the problem and the theoretical orientation. The concept of felt need was considered most appropriate for this study, since the research concentrated on how mothers experienced the problems of caring for a handicapped child. Felt needs are those subjectively experienced by the individuals involved in the situation rather than needs assessed by supposedly objective observers. In decisions about the future of the handicapped child, mothers are likely to be influenced by needs *they feel*, whether or not these are also identified as needs by social workers, doctors, teachers, etc. Thus if a mother feels she needs someone to look after her handicapped child until 5 o'clock every day so that she can go out to work, this may be an important factor in the decision to seek long-term care for the child, and it is irrelevant whether or not a social worker or teacher defines this as an important need. Too often, evaluation of the needs of families caring for a mentally handicapped child is undertaken by people who do not have a full understanding of the problems experienced by those who carry the burden. This can result on the one hand in a failure to identify needs which are felt by family members, and on the other hand in identifying needs which are not considered important by those most involved.

The method of assessing mothers' felt needs for additional support was discussed in Chapter 3. To recapitulate briefly, mothers were asked, for each of the tasks of child care and housework, whether they would like more help than they received at present and, if so, how important they felt it would be to have this additional support. The word' like', rather than 'need', was used because it was found in pilot interviews that mothers were not inclined to identify 'need' if they were actually coping with the situation, however marginally and with whatever difficulties. Thus, for example, a mother who complained that her handicapped child drove her crazy during the school holidays said, when asked whether she needed extra help in the holidays, that she could manage. However, when asked whether she would like additional help she said that she most certainly would and that such help would make a very important difference to her. All mothers in the study were, by definition, coping with their handicapped child, and the level of need reported was thus very low, since all the mothers could manage without extra help. They were defining needs according to minimum standards, perhaps taking their cue from what appears to be social services policy; i.e. that anything short of crisis does not represent need. Since the implicit assumption behind this research was that support may be able to prevent crises, the questions were rephrased from: 'Do you need more help?' to 'Would you like more help?', so that situations that had not yet reached desperation would be included in the positive answers. However, a further qualification was necessary since it was clear that mothers attached more importance to having help with some tasks than with others. Accordingly, they were asked to rate the degree of importance attached to having additional support with each individual task as 'not very important', 'important' or 'very important'. The rating of the degree of importance attached to having more help was left entirely up to the mothers, since the objective was to establish what they felt about child care and housework. In practice the gradings worked well, mothers identifying some tasks with which, although they would have liked additional support, this support would not have made a crucial difference to them, and other tasks in which the availability of additional help would have made a most important difference to their ability to cope with the situation. In order to obtain overall assessments of the levels of felt need, responses to the questions were scored on a four point scale and the scores for each item were added to produce an overall index of need. At the extremes, a mother who expressed no desire for more help with a particular task scored 0, whilst one who wanted more help and rated such help as very important scored 3. Separate scores were calculated for tasks in each of the three groups; physical child care, child minding and housework. Since the main concern was with mothers' subjective interpretations, no attempt was made to give differential weightings to tasks, other than those provided by the mothers themselves in the degree of importance attached to having more help. Thus the scores obtained using this procedure are comparative rather than absolute, so that a high level of need is only relative to lower levels reported by other mothers in the study.

Felt needs for additional support are analysed in three different ways in this chapter. First, the felt needs of all mothers for support with individual tasks are considered in order to provide an impression of the numbers of mothers who would have welcomed help with each task. In addition, scores for each group of tasks (physical child care, child minding, housework) are presented, in order to provide an idea of the relative importance of additional support with different types of tasks. The tables in each of these sections refer to the unmatched groups, since the objective was to examine the extent to which mothers of severely mentally handicapped children as a whole felt the need for extra help. Secondly, there follows a discussion of the relationship between felt needs and the decision to seek long-term care for the handicapped child. The ways in which mothers perceived their circumstances and the extent to which they felt the need for additional support might be expected to have considerable bearing upon whether or not they felt it necessary to seek long-term care. The data presented in this discussion refers only to the matched groups, since it is necessary to look at differences in the levels of felt need between groups who faced simlar objective situations in terms of the age and degree of handicap of the child. Thirdly, the relationship between levels of felt need and mothers' expectations for their own lives is considered. The argument is advanced that mothers who expressed high levels of need tended to belong to families in which there was a tendency to be dissatisfied with existing conditions and to aspire to an improved quality of life. The chapter concludes with a discussion of the importance of felt needs for the development of services for the mentally handicapped and their families.

Felt Needs of all the Mothers

Physical Child Care

Table 8.1

Task	No help wanted	Not very important	Important	Very important	Total (100%)
Dressing and undressing children	62 (77%)	0	10 (12%)	9 (11%)	81
Washing and bathing children	97 (84%)	4 (3%)	9 (8%)	6 (5%)	116
Changing nappies	54 (76%)	4 (6%)	7 (10%)	6 (9%)	71
Taking children to toilet	60 (94%)	0	4 (6%)	0	64
Feeding or supervising children at meal-times	81 (85%)	5 (5%)	8 (8%)	1 (1%)	95
Lifting and carrying children	43 (69%)	0	10 (16%)	9 (15%)	62

Table 8.1 shows, for each of the six tasks of physical child care, the numbers of mothers who said they would like more help and how important they felt it was to have this extra help. For each task, those mothers who did not have a child who required the task performing were excluded, so, for example, there were only 71 mothers who had a child in nappies. Children other than the handicapped child were included since they were sometimes just as much of a strain on the mothers' resources. Only relatively small proportions of mothers said they wanted more help with any of the physical aspects of child care. Only 17 mothers, for example, wanted more help with changing nappies and only 6 of these felt that such extra help would have been very important. In many families physical child care, particularly of younger children, did not in itself constitute a major burden, but there was a considerable minority in which physical care was very difficult. Nevertheless, some of the mothers in this latter category did not express a need for additional support. It appeared that they accepted physical care as an essential part of their roles as mothers. Most accepted that physical care was something for which they should be responsible and which, in any case, they felt they were better able to do than others. They did not identify these tasks as in themselves restricting and did not therefore feel that extra help would have made a very great difference to their lives. Of course, this is not to say that increased involvement of other family members would have been rejected had it been

offered.

The fact that the overall level of need expressed in relation to these tasks was low should not, however, obscure the importance of particular problems in particular situations. There were a total of 31 instances in which additional support, had it been available would have been regarded as a very important contribution to the domestic routine. Of the 19 mothers who wanted more help with lifting and carrying the handicapped child 9 regarded this as very important. Most of us might not identify lifting and carrying as a major problem warranting special attention and indeed, for the majority of mothers, this was a fair assessment, but in specific circumstances the problems could constitute a major disruption of the domestic routine. For some of these mothers this had become such a problem that it was a major factor in the decision to apply for admission to long-term care of the handicapped child. In one family, a 14-year-old chair-fast child had to sleep in the living room because there was nobody to help him upstairs. His mother had given up trying to lift him since she had developed severe back pains. Advice about appropriate methods of lifting her child, minor housing alterations, rehousing or the provision of mechanical aids might have considerably eased this mother's problems. Other mothers found dressing and undressing their handicapped child very difficult. Of the 19 who wanted more help with this, 9 felt that it would have made an important difference to them. In some cases 30 minutes to one hour had to be allowed each morning for dressing. Help from other family members and the opportunity to discuss such difficulties with someone who might be able to suggest more effective ways of coping with the problem (e.g. teachers) might have made the lives of these mothers much easier. The fact that these problems were not experienced by large numbers of mothers, and were not therefore likely to attract the attention of those who plan services, does not mean that they were not important for the families concerned.

Table 8.2: Felt Need for Additional Support with Physical Child Care Tasks by Social Age of Handicapped Child

| Felt need for additional support | Social age | | | | |
	1 yr	1-2 yrs	2 -4 yrs	4 yrs	Total
Low	13 (38%)	15 (54%)	30 (83%)	20 (91%)	78 (65%)
Medium	12 (35%)	7 (25%)	3 (8%)	1 (5%)	23 (19%)
High	9 (27%)	6 (21%)	3 (8%)	1 (5%)	19 (16%)
Total (100%)	34	28	36	11	120

Problems of physical care are clearly related to the handicapped child's level of development; the greater a child's capacity for self-care the fewer the problems. Table 8.2 illustrates the relationship between expressed need for additional support with physical child care and the child's social age (as measured by the Vineland Social Maturity Scale). Not surprisingly, the largest proportion of mothers who reported a high level of need, when scores on individual items were amalgamated to produce an overall index, was found to be among those with children with a social age of below one year. Of these mothers, 62 per cent expressed a medium or high level of need compared with only 9 per cent of those with a child having a social age of four years or above. There was a simple gradient with social age, the higher the child's level of development the less likely the mother was to feel the need for additional support with physical care, although many of the care tasks were still applicable. Most of the mothers who expressed a high level of need for support with physical child care had handicapped children who were over five years of age but whose social age was below that of the average one year old. It was thus the context in which physical care had to be given that influenced the levels of felt need for additional support. The problems tended not to take on a special significance until the child had passed well beyond the age at which he or she might be expected to have become independent in these things, and problems of physical size also became more and more difficult to cope with. It might be possible for the services to do more to help such families by devoting special attention to those whose child is, say, over seven years of age with a level of development below that of the average two year old. The important thing is to make sure that advice and practical support are available at an early stage before the situation has become impossible to cope with.

Child Minding

The levels of need expressed in relation to child minding tasks shown in Table 8.3 are in marked contrast to those expressed in relation to physical aspects of child care. Whilst mothers largely accepted the burden of physically caring for their handicapped child, a large proportion wanted some help with tasks under the heading of minding.

When all these tasks were combined to produce an overall score, in the same way as for physical care tasks, 80 per cent of mothers expressed medium or high levels of need compared with only 35 per cent for physical child-care tasks. The tasks with which the largest proportion of mothers wanted more help were looking after children during the school holidays, at weekends and baby sitting. As many as 48 per cent said that help in the school holidays would have made a very important difference to them. School holidays were one of the most difficult times for the mothers and, the problem of providing some form of care at this time for the children warrants serious attention on the part of the services. For many mothers, the school holidays, when they were alone with the handicapped child every day for a number of weeks, were anticipated with horror, and it was no exaggeration when some of them described themselves as prisoners in their own homes. Almost half of them also expressed the need for more help at weekends and with baby sitting. They were asking for the right to lead what they, and most other people, regard as normal lives. They wanted to be able to go out in the evenings and to relax and pursue recreational activities with the rest of the family at weekends. Although holidays, weekends and baby sitting were regarded as most important, a considerable minority of mothers also expressed the need for help in minding children after school and for longer school hours. Most of those who wanted more help at these times did so because they wanted to go out to work but were unable to find work which would fit in with the limited hours the child was at school. Although many had financial reasons for wanting to go out to work, social reasons were often just as important. Many felt terribly isolated and, unlike most mothers of normal children who might expect more freedom as the children grow older, they could see little prospect of an improvement in their circumstances.

Table 8.3: Felt Need for Additional Support with Minding Children

Task	No extra help wanted	Not very important	Important	Very important	Total (100%)
Day care	77 (64%)	8 (7%)	16 (13%)	19 (16%)	120
Minding children after school	86 (72%)	2 (2%)	17 (14%)	15 (13%)	120
Minding children at weekends	62 (52%)	5 (4%)	22 (18%)	31 (26%)	120
Minding children in school holidays	38 (32%)	4 (3%)	21 (18%)	57 (48%)	120
Baby sitting	65 (54%)	8 (7%)	17 (14%)	30 (25%)	120

Table 8.4: Felt Need for Additional Support with Child Minding by Handicapped Child's Social Age

Felt need for additional support	< 1 yr	Social age 1-2 yrs	2-4 yrs	4 yrs	Total
Low	3 (9%)	5 (18%)	9 (25%)	6 (27%)	23 (19%)
Medium	5 (15%)	9 (32%)	10 (28%)	7 (32%)	31 (26%)
High	26 (77%)	14 (50%)	17 (47%)	9 (41%)	66 (55%)
Total (100%)	34	38	36	22	120

The relationship between levels of felt need in relation to child minding tasks and the social age of the handicapped child (Table 8.4) is similar to that shown in relation to physical care tasks, except that the proportion of mothers expressing a high level of need is higher in all categories. At the extremes, 77 per cent of mothers with a child with a social age of one year or below expressed a high level of need compared with 41 per cent of those whose child had a social age of four years or more. The level of expressed need was closely related to the severity of the child's handicap, and thus to the practical problems experienced. Although no comparable data was available for 'normal' families, it is likely that many mothers would express a legitimate desire for more help with looking after children. Thus, although the gradient shown in Table 8.4 would be likely to continue with the increasing social age of the child, it is apparent from the proportion of mothers expressing high levels of need in the higher social age categories that it levels off. It is possible that mothers of the least severely handicapped children in this sample expressed a level of felt need for additional support with child minding which was only slightly higher than that felt by mothers who do not have a handicapped child. The difference, of course, is that these mothers did not have much prospect of their child achieving complete independence and therefore of releasing them from some of their responsibilities.

The high level of felt need in relation to child minding as compared to physical care suggests that mothers regarded it as important to be relieved of the responsibility for tasks rather than only being helped. It was not uncommon for them to say: 'If you're there then you may as well do it yourself.' To have someone help with changing nappies or dressing the handicapped child may be useful, but to have someone look after the children during the holidays or to baby-sit in the evenings actually releases the mother to be able to do something else or just relax without responsibilities. This sort of help could, in part, have been

provided by other family members, but there was also a need for
support from outside the family, either through informal channels or
from the services. Of the 26 mothers who expressed a high level of need
and whose child was profoundly handicapped (social age below one
year), 21 had a relatively high level of support from other members of
their families. But having support only from a husband or other
children was often unsatisfactory, since it still failed to release the
mothers to do the things they wanted to do. For example, the fact that
a husband was prepared to baby-sit was of little use if the mother
wanted to go out with her husband. In order to provide an effective
network of support it is essential to utilise different sources, including
the services, but the latter must be sufficiently flexible to take account
of the needs of individual families and their existing patterns of support.

Household Tasks

Table 8.5: Felt Need for Additional Support with Household tasks

Task	No extra help wanted	Not very important	Important	Very important	Total (100%)
Cleaning and tidying the house	98 (82%)	3 (3%)	9 (8%)	9 (8%)	120
Cooking and preparing meals	115 (96%)	1 (1%)	1 (1%)	3 (3%)	120
Washing dishes and laying the table	115 (96%)	4 (3%)	1 (1%)	0	120
Washing and ironing clothes	103 (86%)	3 (3%)	11 (9%)	3 (3%)	120
Shopping	108 (90%)	2 (2%)	7 (6%)	3 (3%)	120
Transport	59 (49%)	7 (6%)	18 (15%)	38 (32%)	120

The difficulties some mothers had in getting through the daily grind of
household chores were described in Chapter 5. The handicapped child
often created extra housework in the form of cleaning and washing
clothes, and sometimes further complicated matters by refusing to
allow the mother to get on with the work. These problems seemed to
be further compounded by the fact that their husbands and other
children did little to help with housework, but in spite of these difficulties the level of expressed need for additional support with household tasks was generally low (Table 8.5). Very few mothers saw the
availability of more help with housework as a solution to their
problems. Only five attached any importance to having extra help with

cooking and preparing meals, and assistance with washing and ironing clothes, which was often a very demanding task, was felt to be important by only seven mothers. There seem to be two likely explanations for this relatively low level of felt need. First, most mothers consciously accepted a domestic division of labour, in which jobs such as washing and cooking were clearly delineated obligations of the maternal role. To have expressed a general desire for additional help with housework would have been to admit that they had failed to live up to their expectations of themselves. Where they did want more help it was often related to a specific problem. For example, those mothers who wanted more help with shopping either had a child whose behaviour (e.g. grabbing items off supermarket shelves or screaming) made shopping impossible, or they lived some distance from the shops with a severely physically disabled child and no means of transport. Almost all the mothers who wanted more help with washing clothes had doubly incontinent children and some had no washing machine or dryer. It seemed that the presence of such specific and obvious problems enabled mothers to feel that it was not a sign of failure to ask for help. The second reason for the low level of expressed need for additional support with housework was probably at least as important as the desire to perform their maternal roles to the satisfaction of themselves and other people. Such support, unlike help with child minding, would not have released them to do other things. To have had their husbands help with cooking meals, for instance, would not have enabled them to get out more or to go out to work.

No mention has so far been made in this section of the last item in Table 8.5 – transport. It is included with household tasks for the sake of convenience, although in many ways it constitutes a separate category. Mothers were asked if they would like any help getting to and from places. Over half regarded transport as a problem and wanted more help with it. In some cases, getting a severely disabled 14- or 15-year-old to the bus stop and then managing to get him or her on and off the bus totally defeated them. In other cases, the physical problems could be overcome but mothers found that their child either refused to get on or, once on the bus, refused to get off again. If mothers had received more help with transport problems when the handicapped child was at home they would have found activities such as shopping, visiting friends, going on day trips, etc. so much easier. In this respect, help with transport was in the same category as help with child minding, in that it would have enabled them to do things that they were otherwise prevented from doing. One mother had been forced to abandon visiting her elderly parents because, since her handicapped child could not be persuaded to go on a bus, the only way she could get there was by taxi. For those who found that the only way to overcome the problem was to go everywhere on foot, the saving in time that would have been achieved through having some help with transport would have been enormous. However, it should be noted that, since this study was completed, many families have become eligible for a mobility allowance which has done much to ease the problems. In the light of the large numbers of mothers in this study who wanted help with transport it is most important to make sure that families are aware that they are eligible for the allowance and to assist them in making applications.

Felt Needs and the Decision to Institutionalise — Comparison of Groups Matched for Age and Social Quotient

Table 8.6: Felt Need for Additional Support with Child Minding (Scores) by Group (Age and SQ Matched)

Felt need for additional support	Group		
	Home	Admissions	Total
Low	7 (23%)	3 (10%)	10 (17%)
Medium	12 (40%)	5 (17%)	17 (28%)
High	11 (37%)	22 (73%)	33 (55%)
Total (100%)	30	30	60

Table 8.7: Felt Need for Additional Support (Child Care and Household Tasks) Overall Scores by Group (Matched for Age and SQ)

Felt need for additional support	Group		
	Home	Social worker referrals	Total
Low	4 (13%)	2 (7%)	6 (10%)
Medium	18 (60%)	11 (37%)	29 (48%)
High	8 (27%)	17 (57%)	25 (42%)
Total (100%)	30	30	60

The decision to seek long-term care for a severely mentally handicapped child, although very much influenced by the objective circumstances in which a family finds itself, is ultimately a reflection of how family members, and the mother in particular, feel about these circumstances. In general, mothers whose child was awaiting admission to long-term care expressed a much higher level of felt need for additional support than did those in the home group, but Table 8.6 shows that there was a particularly sharp contrast between the groups in the levels of felt need in respect of child minding tasks. Whilst 73 per cent of admissions group mothers expressed a high level of need for help with these tasks this was true of only 37 per cent of home group mothers. The pattern was similar in relation to physical child-care tasks and household tasks but, as a consequence of the generally lower level of felt need for additional support in these areas, the differences between the two groups were much less pronounced. It was suggested earlier that the generally higher level of felt need for support with child minding compared with other tasks reflected the fact that such support would have enabled the mothers to spend time on activities which were otherwise impossible. Those in the admissions group consistently stressed the importance of such support. When all tasks were combined to produce an overall index of the level of felt need for additional support (Table 8.7), 57 per cent of admissions group mothers had high scores compared with only 27 per cent of those in the home group.

These differences between the two groups in terms of felt needs can be explained in a number of ways. First and foremost, they suggest that mothers in the admissions group were less likely to accept their situation and were therefore more likely to ask for the sort of help which would have eased the problems. This in turn suggests that the way in which they perceived the situation might have been an important factor in the decision as to whether long-term should be sought for the handicapped child. Those mothers who saw themselves in terms other than their purely domestic roles seemed much more likely to opt for long-term care since this was, in practice, the only way in which they could hope to be able to spend some of their time on activities outside the home. However, there were two other factors which may have accounted for at least part of the difference between the two groups. First, more of the handicapped children in the admissions group presented severe behaviour problems and mothers of such children were more likely to express the need for additional support, particularly with child minding tasks. Analysis of the data on behavioural problems though, indicated that these only accounted for a relatively small proportion of the difference between the two groups. The second possible explanation of the higher level of need reported by mothers in the admissions group is that this was a reflection of rationalisations that had been made *since* the decision to seek long-term care was taken. It is conceivable that, in expressing a high level of need, mothers were attempting to justify the decision to seek long-term care by stressing the problems of keeping the child at home. The only way to establish whether or not this process could explain the difference between the two groups would be to carry out a longitudinal study of families, beginning before any such decisions had been taken. However, it seems unlikely that this process of justification could account for the large differences observed, although it is possible that mothers found it easier to admit the needs and desires to pursue other activities once the traumatic decision to seek long-term care had been taken. The realisation of limitations imposed by the handicapped child may become much easier when the alternatives become a real possibility. It may be easier, for example, for a mother to admit that she would like to go out to work when she knows that the handicapped child will soon go into long-term care and that she will then have the opportunity to choose how she spends her time.

Even allowing for the fact that there are various possible explanations for differences between the groups in levels of felt needs, the information available from the study suggests that mothers' feelings about their circumstances were of crucial importance in the relationship between needs and the decision to seek long-term care. Earlier chapters have shown that differences in the circumstances of families and the levels of support received by mothers were relatively small, and often slightly in favour of those families in the admissions group. In particular, these families received somewhat better services, but the mothers interpreted these circumstances in a very different way from the home group mothers. The measurement of need through objective criteria such as the degree of handicap, level of income, housing accommodation and size of family is an important element in understanding why families seek long-term care, but these objective facts are interpreted by individuals in different ways. Their subjective interpretations form the basis on which decisions are ultimately taken and, as such, require careful consideration by policy-makers and those responsible for providng services to families. In order to respond to the needs of families, and mothers in particular, the services must be aware not only of the objective circumstances, but also of how individuals feel about these. It must be appreciated that economic and social changes over a period of time lead to changes in the perceptions that people have. Care of the severely mentally handicapped in the community must be based on a partnership between families and services in which the latter are closely in touch with the needs of families and are making every effort to meet these, rather than allowing families to cope alone until the only way that their needs can be met is by taking the painful decision to ask for the child's admission to long-term care.

Needs and Expectations

Mothers' expectations for their own lives have been referred to a
number of times in earlier chapters and it has been suggested that the
extent to which they felt themselves restricted by the handicapped child
was an important factor in determining whether or not to seek institutional care for the child. In particular it was shown that mothers in
the admissions group were more likely than those in the home group to
want to go out to work, to have more free time and to go out more in
the evenings. Seeking long-term care, however, was only one way in
which they might have overcome these restrictions. Longer hours of day
care, provisions for the school holidays, a baby-sitting service, etc. might
also have enabled the mothers to have overcome the restrictions. Since
such services were not available, it was not surprising that those mothers
who wanted to go out to work, have more leisure time, etc. expressed a
much higher level of need for additional help than did those who were
more accepting of their circumstances (Tables 8.8 to 8.10). There
appeared to be differences in mothers' attitudes towards the maternal
role and the obligations associated with it. The comprehensive care of a
severely mentally handicapped child often requires nothing less than
devotion on the part of the person bearing the major responsibility.
Many mothers who talked to the interviewers expressed this sort of
devotion, often saying that they lived for their handicapped child. They
obtained a sense of fulfilment through caring for him or her and from
completing the daily round of routine domestic chores. There was no
question for these mothers of seeking residential care for their child, at
least in the foreseeable future. They saw themselves as wives and
mothers, and were content to derive their status from fulfilling, to the
best of their abilities, the arduous duties of caring for their family and
their handicapped child. To the extent that they expressed needs for
more support and felt their activities were restricted, these were usually
connected with activities which also involved the handicapped child.
Mrs Barnet said: 'I have no particular difficulties with Alan. I'd like to
be able to buy him more clothes and to get away with Alan for a good
holiday, but it's not financially possible.

However, these mothers were in a minority, since the role of women
as domestic servants is increasingly being questioned by women themselves. Mrs Walters wanted to go out to work, even if only part-time:
'My husband thinks I've got enough to do with Helen and all the housework, but I get bored and lonely being at home all day long on my
own.' Many of the mothers interviewed expressed a desire to go out to
work, to develop social relationships, to make use of entertainment

Table 8.8: Felt Need for Additional Support (Overall Scores) by Whether Mothers Would Like to Go Out to Work or Work Longer Hours

	Like to go out to work		
Felt needs	Yes	No	Total
Low	2 (3%)	9 (19%)	11 (10%)
Medium	36 (54%)	21 (45%)	59 (52%)
High	29 (43%)	15 (32%)	44 (39%)
Total (100%)	67	47	114

Table 8.9: Felt Need for Additional Support (overall Scores) by Whether Mothers Would Like to Go Out More in the Evenings

	Like to go out more		
Felt Needs	Yes	No	Total
Low	5 (7%)	7 (14%)	12 (10%)
Medium	28 (41%)	33 (67%)	61 (52%)
High	36 (52%)	9 (18%)	45 (38%)
Total (100%)	69	49	118

Table 8.10: Felt Need for Additional Support (Overall Scores) by Whether Mothers Would Like More Time at Weekends

	Like more time at weekend		
Felt Needs	Yes	No	Total
Low	5 (6%)	7 (18%)	12 (10%)
Medium	37 (46%)	24 (62%)	61 (51%)
High	38 (48%)	8 (21%)	46 (39%)
Total (100%)	80	39	119

facilities, to take up hobbies, etc. For some these were seen as predominantly family-oriented activities, but for others they were a means of developing their own independence. On the one hand Mrs Evans stressed family-centred activities: 'I'd like us to be able to do more as a family just to spend more time together. I'd like to be able to take the children out or to the zoo.' In contrast Mrs Newman emphasised the importance of independent activities: 'I'd like to be able to go out to work and meet a few people, to have a good laugh and bring me out of myself. I'd like to go dancing and go to concerts, things like that.'

In these things mothers of severely mentally handicapped children are no different from many other women, except that the restrictions that surround them are often more difficult to overcome. In our society the nuclear family is becoming smaller and kinship networks are smaller and often geographically more distant than they were in the past. If a woman expects her life to revolve around the family and her social identity to be defined in terms of the family, the limitations imposed by the presence of a severely mentally handicapped child may be manageable, but for many women, the family is no longer seen as an institution which can meet all their legitimate needs. It is hardly surprising that some of these mothers of mentally handicapped children, like other women, were looking for opportunities to become more involved in life outside the family. Conversely, however, others wanted more time free from responsibilities of caring for a mentally handicapped child so that they could better full women's traditional roles in the family.

In a more general way, the expression of needs and expectations by mothers reflected a rejection of the view that their circumstances were unalterable. Whilst there were some families in which the mother said: 'It's my cross to bear' or 'God gave me this child to look after', there were many others who were striving to improve thier lives in all sorts of ways. Our society emphasises individual achievements, claims that people have the ability to control and change circumstances, and continually flaunts, through the media, the high standard of living that some people have. It is hardly surprising, therefore, that many people express dissatisfaction with conditions which are far from the ideals that are presented to them. Table 8.11 suggests that this expression of needs was related to the social group from which the mothers came. The level of need expressed by mothers in social classes IV and V was lower than that expressed by others although, in terms of material conditions, they were probably worse off. This suggests a possible polarisation of families into the two categories which Susser and Watson called aspirant and demotic.[1] The aspirant family is more likely to express dissatisfaction with existing conditions and to strive to change and improve these conditions, whereas the demotic family may be characterised as much more accepting of the status quo. One might expect the aspirant families to be more commonly found in social classes II and III, and it was true that families in these groups were more likely to express a high level of felt need. In turn it can be suggested that aspirant families were more likely than demotic families to seek long-term institutional care for their handicapped child, since they tended to perceive the child as an obstacle to improving the overall conditions of life. This is one more factor which may throw light on the question of why some families

Table 8.11: Felt Need for Additional Support (Child Care and Household Tasks) Overall Scores by Social Class

| Felt Needs | Social Class | | | |
	I, II, III non-manual	III manual	IV and V	Total
Low	2 (13%)	1 (3%)	6 (12%)	9
Medium	6 (40%)	16 (44%)	28 (57%)	50
High	7 (47%)	19 (53%)	15 (30%)	41
Total	15	36	49	100

seek long-term care whilst others do not.

Discussion

The data that has been discussed in this chapter highlights the importance of the concept of felt need in decisions relating to the long-term
hospital or residential care of the handicapped child, and therefore its
importance for the way in which services for the mentally handicapped
and their families should be developed. But needs, however defined,
cannot be viewed in a static way. The preceding discussion has tried to
relate the felt needs expressed by mothers in this study to changes taking
place within society as a whole. The feelings reported by some mothers
of handicapped children reflect generally changing attitudes about the
role of women, and the part that child care, housework, the family, etc.
should play in their lives. It is likely that in the future more mothers
will perceive and seek to change sources of dissatisfaction in their lives.
This is not to suggest that they will wish to put away their handicapped
children at the earliest opportunity. On the contrary, both the mothers
and the professionals usually want the child to remain at home for as
long as possible, but to facilitate this, account will have to be taken of
changing attitudes and expectations. The effective pursual of a policy of
community care depends upon a realistic appraisal of how care in the
family operates, how families, and particularly mothers, feel about it
and what changes are likely to affect patterns of caring and attitudes in
the future. Earlier chapters in this report have documented the day-to-
day reality of what community care implies for mothers and this
chapter has concentrated on how mothers feel about this in terms of
their felt needs for more support than they already receive.

In terms of specific services for which there is already a widely felt
need, this chapter has identified a number of important areas. The large
majority of mothers emphasised the importance of support which

would relieve them of responsibilities for some periods and therefore enable them to engage in other activities. In terms of the order of importance attached to them by mothers the following areas would seem to warrant immediate attention:

1. Provision of some form of day care during the school holidays.
2. Longer school hours or alternative provisions after school.
3. Day care or play facilities for some time at weekends.
4. Some form of baby-sitting service or the development of voluntary babysitting groups.
5. Some form of help with transport problems.

These will receive more discussion in the following chapter with specific suggestions as to possibilities for meeting these needs. However, these are only the areas in which large numbers of mothers expressed the need for additional support. It has been stressed throughout the discussion of needs that, although only small numbers of mothers reported needs in many task areas, this should not lead to a neglect of these problems merely because they are not felt by large numbers of people. The heterogeneous nature of the severely mentally handicapped as a group means that the problems experienced in caring for them are extremely varied. The fact that only nine mothers felt that more help with lifting and carrying their handicapped child would be very important should not mean that these problems are ignored. In particular situations particular problems can be crucial in making the difference between being able to cope and not being able to cope. Beyond the four areas of need which were felt by a large proportion of mothers, most needs were highly individual, but nevertheless important. If support for mothers with a mentally handicapped child is to be effective, then it must be developed in such a way that it is able to identify the problems and deal with them in a flexible way which takes account of individual circumstances.

9 CONCLUSIONS

It is customary at this point in a book describing a piece of research to emphasise the limitations of the research methodology and, therefore, the caution necessary in drawing conclusions from the findings. It is true that the samples used in this study were relatively small, drawn from particular geographical areas and that the scope of the research was limited, thus excluding many relevant questions. It is also true that the sample of families whose child was awaiting admission to long-term residential care was selected in such a way that makes it difficult to assess whether or not it was representative of all children being admitted to long-term residential care. Nevertheless, the need for caution in drawing conclusions should not be over-emphasised. The main conclusions are strongly supported by evidence from this research and by the experience of many field workers who have long experience of working with the mentally handicapped and their families. There are in fact good grounds for supposing that the samples used in this study were representative of similar populations in other parts of the country. The administrative definition of severe mental handicap is the same in all parts of this country; economic, cultural and social conditions do not vary greatly, and, whilst there are variations in the level of service provisions from one area to another, the basic structure of services is the same. Thus, whilst the reader should bear in mind any specific local circumstances, in general, the conclusions of this study are likely to be applicable to the vast majority of families with a severely mentally handicapped child in other parts of the country. Finally in this context, it should be remembered that the interviews were conducted during 1974 and 1975. This means, on the one hand, that there have been improvements in services for the mentally handicapped and their families, although in most areas these improvements have been painfully slow. On the other hand, however, it is likely that the processes of social change described have continued to create increased needs for services.

In this final chapter the most important findings of the study are summarised, and from these findings conclusions are drawn concerning the care of severely mentally handicapped children in the future. These conclusions are considered under three headings: the nuclear family; informal metworks of support; and the services, since these three elements make up the structure of community care. The services for the mentally handicapped and their families are the element most amenable to planning, and their future development is considered in the context of changes in the family and the community. The discussion of services contains both specific recommendations for improvements in existing services and more general comments on the organisation and structure of services and the ways in which they should be developed. Whilst existing services leave much to be desired, a number of recent improvements which provide grounds for cautious optimism are discussed. Finally, these conclusions are placed in their overall economic and political context, since the mentally handicapped are only one of many groups fighting for scarce economic resources.

The Main Findings

The Handicapped Children

It is worth repeating a point which was made at the very beginning of this book: mental handicap is a diverse condition with a wide range of causes and associated mental, physical and social problems. Severe mental handicap is a convenient administrative label, but it fails to convey much meaning, other than that people so labelled suffer a considerable degree of mental impairment. The children in this study ranged from the profoundly handicapped who were unable even to sit up, to those who were on the border line of mild mental handicap. There were sharp contrasts, however, between children who were awaiting admission to long-term care (the admissions group) and those who were not (the home group), in their ages, the severity of their physical and mental handicaps and the number of severe behaviour problems they presented. The likelihood of admission to long-term care increases as the child grows older, so that 81 per cent of admissions group children were over eight years of age compared with 58 per cent of those in the home group. Whilst age was obviously an important factor, the overall level of social maturity seemed even more critical. In spite of their greater average chronological age, 44 per cent of admissions group children had social ages of below one year, compared with only 7 per cent of home group children. Similarly, the presence of behaviour problems often made the difference between being able to cope and having to seek long-term care; 44 per cent of children awaiting admission presented five or more marked problems in contrast to only 15 per cent of those in the home group. Thus it was clear that age, severity of handicap and behaviour problems were major factors in the decision to seek long-term residential care. Nevertheless, there was a considerable number of children *not* awaiting admission who had many of the same characteristics as those who were. Whilst the characteristics of the handicapped child constitute a major element in the equation leading to the decision to seek long-term care, one must look beyond these to establish why some families continue to manage the child at home whereas others find similar problems impossible to cope with.

The Families

The mentally handicapped children came from a wide variety of back-grounds, reflecting the fact that the incidence of severe mental handicap is not related to social class. In addition, and perhaps more surprisingly, there was no relationship between the social class and whether or not the family was seeking long-term care. This was not true, however, with regard to family structure. This did make a difference since, of the nine one-parent families, seven were in the home group, which also contained more large families. One might have expected that large families and fatherless families would find the problems of coping with the handicapped child more difficult, but this did not seem to be the case. There was no appreciable difference between the groups in the proportion of fathers who were unemployed. In fact it was high in both groups (18 per cent) which suggests that long-term unemployment may be one strategy employed by some families to cope with the burdens of caring for a handicapped child. Information was collected about the mothers and their reactions to the problems of caring for their child. Compared with mothers in the home group, those whose child was awaiting admission were slightly younger, experienced more problems with their physical and mental health and were more likely to express resentment at being unable to go out to work or to enjoy satisfactory social lives. The mothers' state of health and feelings about the restrictions they experienced as a result of caring for their handicapped child were probably the most important family factors having a bearing on the decision to seek long-term care.

The Daily Routine

A detailed study of the daily domestic routine in the home was under-taken, since it was considered that any attempts to describe community care would be meaningless without the careful analysis of the routine activities that comprise family care of a severely mentally handicapped child. The burdens of child care and housework were largely carried by mothers with little or no support from any source. Rather than referring to 'community care' or 'family care', it would be more accurate to refer to 'maternal care', since this was the reality in most families. In the light of the very low level of support that most mothers received, it was perhaps not surprising that there were no major differences between the two groups in the levels of support that mothers received. This should not be taken to imply that support with the domestic routine has no bearing on the likelihood that a family will seek institutional care, merely that current levels of support are so low as to be irrelevant. Consequently, It was found that other factors were more likely to account for the families' decisions as to whether or not to keep the child at home.

Informal Support

Informal support refers to that provided by other family members, relatives, friends and neighbours. The help that mothers received was very low in relation to the amount of work necessary, but nevertheless, the study recorded who provided the help that was available and who might have done more to help. Support from within the family was very limited and certainly not sufficient to justify the description of 'family care'; support from outside the family was, in most case, virtually non-existent. Fathers were the greatest single source of support but they provided much less help than they might have done. Their contribution (only 25 per cent had a high level of participation in child care and housework) reflected a very traditional division of labour in the home; the mothers being responsible for the children and the home whilst their husbands went out to work. The fact that all these families had a highly dependent child appeared to make no difference to the involvement of most fathers in routine child care and household tasks. Similarly, siblings of the handicapped child rarely made a major contribution to the domestic routine, but where they did, their help was extremely valuable, although necessarily temporary, since most of them were growing up and would leave home within a few years. Relatives provided little direct support with aspects of the domestic routine, although a large proportion lived sufficiently close to the families and saw them sufficiently often to have been able to provide some support. Thus the notion of a close supportive kinship network was not a reality for most of these families. Similarly, they were unable to rely on help from friends or neighbours with routine tasks; a number of families did not have even one neighbour of whom they felt they could ask a favour.

The Services

Only education and short-term residential care provided large numbers of families with the sort of support that had a major impact on their day-to-day routines, and therefore on their ability to cope with the handicapped child. Most mothers spoke appreciatively of the schools, but there were a number of criticisms, the most common of which were the lack of opportunity for discussion with the teachers and the difficult and often unreliable arrangements for bussing the children to school. Compliments were, unfortunately, less common in respect of the health services. Mothers' experiences with doctors were extremely varied and usually dependent on the level of knowledge and understanding about the problem that the doctors possessed. Those mothers who had the good fortune to have a doctor who was able to provide information and understand the problems counted themselves very lucky. So many others related experiences with doctors who seemed to know little about handicapped children and to care even less. Social services departments have a very important role to play in providing much needed practical support for families, but in most cases they were failing to fulfil this role. The services they provided seemed to reflect a crisis orientation, in that admissions group families had received much more help than those in the home group. Only when a family declared itself unable to cope any longer did any kind of help seem to be forthcoming. Those services that families did receive also left much to be desired. In particular, non-specialist social workers came in for a great deal of criticism. Mothers complained that they did not know what the social worker was supposed to do and the social worker did not seem to have much idea either. About one third of all families had received some form of help from voluntary agencies of one sort or another. The help they received from these agencies was often of more use than that provided by the statutory services, although it too was somewhat unevenly distributed and sporadic. Finally, two-thirds of the children had received spells of short-term residential care during the preceding year, but once again this was concentrated among the admissions group children. Many mothers complained about the location and standard of the accommodation provided and the bureaucratic arrangements for allocating places.

The predominant orientation of services seemed to be crisis management, rather than the provision of long-term support. As long as families appeared to be coping they were assumed to be alright and not to need any additional support. Only when the family appeared to be in danger of collapsing under the strain, and thus seeking long-term care for the child, did the services consider them worthy of support. By this time, for many families, it was already too late, since the decision to seek long-term care had already been taken. It is not possible to say what the effect of providing more support much earlier would have been for those families whose child was awaiting admission, but it would at least have made things easier and may have delayed the decision to seek long-term care.

Felt Needs

Too little attention has, in the past, been devoted to understanding how those responsible for the day-to-day care of handicapped children feel about the problem and what additional help they would most like. Mothers' felt needs for additional support were shown to be a very important factor in the decision to seek long-term care for the child. Mothers of admission group children tended to express a much higher level of felt need than those in the home group in respect of all aspects of child care and housework. Nevertheless, virtually all mothers experienced some need for additional help. The tasks with which most wanted extra support were minding children in the school holidays (68 per cent), day care at weekends (48 per cent), baby-sitting in the evenings (46 per cent), and transport (51 per cent). These were the tasks with which large proportions of mothers wanted help and they therefore warrant attention on a fairly wide scale, but there was a much less obvious need for support with other tasks, such as changing nappies and cleaning the house. Although only a few mothers expressed a need for this sort of help, it would have made a very great difference to their particular problems. To have met the variety of needs that mothers experienced might have made it easier for them to keep the child at home, which was the expressed wish of the majority, including those whose child was awaiting admission.

The Family with a Mentally Handicapped Child — The Future

The Nuclear Family

The nuclear family (parents and childrem), in spite of wide-scale social changes, remains the framework within which children in our society are reared, and it is therefore the basic caring unit for the vast majority of severely mentally handicapped children. Modern alternatives to the nuclear family, such as communes or collectives, have developed during the last 20 years, but it is extremely unlikely that such schemes will affect anything more than a tiny proportion of the population in the foreseeable future. The increase in the number of divorces suggests that there is a tendency to see marriage as a less permanent institution, but the evidence indicates that the majority of people who obtain divorces re-marry within a few years, therefore the basic structure of the family unit has not changed very much. The decline in the birth rate in recent years suggests that there may be a trend towards smaller families but it is likely that this is only a temporary phenomenon and that a decline in the level of unemployment and an increase in the standard of living will reverse this trend. Finally, slum clearance programmes, new housing developments and increased geographical and social mobility during the past 30 years have produced a steady decline in the number of three generation families (nuclear families plus grandparents) living together or in close proximity. Thus for the foreseeable future the majority of severely mentally handicapped children will be cared for by their parents in two-generation households, and if they have siblings, there are unlikely to be more than one or two of them. In other words there are no signs that any major changes, other than the gradual continuation of existing trends, will affect the composition, structure and standard of living of the majority of families.

Although there are unlikely to be major structural changes in the nuclear family, there are other areas in which changes might be expected to have a considerable impact on the care of the mentally handicapped child in the family. The organisation of family life, in terms of the roles of individual family members inside and outside the home, and the aspirations and expectations of the family and the individuals within it, are important factors affecting family care. It was clear from the present study that, in the majority of families, child care and housework remain almost exclusively maternal obligations. The extent to which fathers participate in the ordinary domestic routine may have altered slightly as a result of the increasing numbers of women in employment, but in terms of its impact on the overall division of labour in the home, the affect of any change is marginal. It is probably outweighed by the fact that other individuals who in the past might have provided support, such as relatives and older children, are now less likely to do so. However, the relatively unchanged position of women in the home is at odds with the changes that have taken place and will continue to do so in their position in the wider society. The fact that large numbers of mothers want to go out to work, to go out more socially and to pursue independent activities, reflects changing attitudes towards the position of women in society, particularly on the part of women themselves. Women's social identity has traditionally

been tied to the family, where they have been expected to obtain fulfilment through family life, but women themselves are increasingly
questioning such assumptions. This is leading to a fundamental contradiction, since they are still required to fulfil obligations which place
severe restrictions on their opportunity to undertake other activities.
For many women this contradiction is at least manageable since, with a
small family, the period of full-time child rearing is fairly short, but for
mothers of severely mentally handicapped children the contradiction is
much more sharply felt. They find themselves more or less permanently
restricted by the necessity of caring for a highly dependent child who
will never grow up. There are a number of ways in which this conflict
can be dealt with. First, the problem can be removed by seeking long-
term residential care for the handicapped child, although this is a
solution that many mothers are unwilling to adopt. Secondly, at the
other extreme, some mothers feel forced to abandon their legitimate
aspirations for a life outside the family, and devote their whole lives to
child care. The third solution, which has yet to be tried, but which
surely would be in the best interests of all concerned, would involve
greatly increasing the amount of support available to mothers. This
could only be achieved through changes in the organisation of familial
roles, the availability of more informal support from outside the family
and the provision of more services.

It would be wrong to suggest that the trend towards an increased
desire for freedom and independence was characteristic of all the
mothers interviewed in this study. Many, particularly those in the older
age groups, did not express a desire to extend their lives outside the
family although this does not imply that they did not experience
problems and restrictions. The predominant orientation of these
mothers was towards family life. Thus the restrictions they felt were in
relation to family activities rather than activities which they might have
wanted to undertake independently of other family members. Additional support would have been welcomed by wives and mothers, rather
than to enable them to do things outside the home. They wanted more
time to play with their other children, go on family outings, prepare
meals and keep the house clean. They did not express a desire to go out
to work, engage in hobbies or mix socially with their own friends. They
did not, in general, experience a conflict between their roles inside and
outside the family and were thus less likely to seek long-term care for
their handicapped child. Nevertheless, the fact that they were not
seeking long-term care should not be taken to imply that they did not
experience problems and did not need support. They were less likely to

complain about their circumstances, but they too experienced many frustrations.

Unfortunately, it seems unlikely that the mothers in this study, and others faced with similar problems, will receive the sort of support from other family members that they need, although it is to be hoped that changing attitudes towards the role of women will eventually permeate through to the home. If the support they need is not forthcoming from within the nuclear family then it will have to be provided from outside, either through informal networks or through the formal services.

Informal Networks

People who advocate a policy of community care for the severely mentally handicapped have laid much store by the existence of supportive communities which operate through informal networks of kin, friends and neighbours. This study has cast considerable doubt on the importance which should be attached to these networks as sources of support with the daily routines of child care and housework. Such a conclusion seems, at first sight, to contradict the findings of a number of studies which have shown that there are many ways in which kinship networks continue to play an important role in industrial societies.[1] Why then did these potential sources of support not seem very relevant to the families studied, and what are likely to be the trends in the future?

As far as the extended family is concerned, the findings of this study did not conflict with the view that the *modified* extended family continues to play an important role in modern societies. Many of the families had a high level of contact with kin and there was often some sort of mutual supportive relationship. What the study did show, however, was that support from the kinship network was not usually relevant to the day-to-day domestic routine. There are a number of reasons for this. Mutually supportive networks were probably based on the presence of women in the home, but the increased involvement of women in the labour force has meant that fewer women spend most of their time at home. Increasing geographical mobility has meant that families have become much more widely scattered and there is therefore less likelihood of contact on a day-to-day basis. This increased geographical mobility is also linked to increased social mobility which may create greater social distance both between and within generations in the extended family. Whilst these factors have reduced the frequency and changed the nature of contact between relatives, other developments have reduced the need for mutually supportive relationships.

General improvements in the standard of living have meant that most families have a much greater degree of security and are therefore less likely to need short-term practical and financial support. The decreasing size of families has meant that the amount of work necessary in the home has declined and the period during which children are dependent is shorter. One consequence of these developments is that, for the majority of families, maintaining contact with kin becomes less of a necessity and more a matter of choice. They are no longer relied upon as part of the day-to-day structure for coping with problems. For families with a severely mentally handicapped child, however, the situation is very different. The long-term dependence of one child in the family makes them exceptional in modern society. Whilst residual kinship networks may be adequate to meet the requirements of the majority of families in a modern industrial society, they are not usually adequate to meet the needs of that minority of families with especially heavy needs. Today such families usually have to seek day-to-day support elsewhere, although in certain communities, where traditional patterns of mutual support on a day-to-day basis continue to exist, these can be invaluable and every effort should be made to ensure that re-housing programmes do not disrupt them.

If kinship networks are not adequate to meet the day-to-day needs of mothers of handicapped children for support, can friendship and neighbourhood networks supply an alternative source of support? Unfortunately, the evidence from this study was that friends provided even less support in day-to-day routines than did relatives. Support of the type considered was not seen as appropriate to the role of friend, and mothers did not in general expect to give or receive such support from their friends. They regarded friends as important in a social and psychological sense but did not see them as being able or willing to provide assistance in meeting day-to-day problems. Similarly, neighbours, other than those who had achieved a satus of friend, played an insignificant part in the lives of most families. The cosy idea of neighbourhood mutual support systems conveyed in the concept of community care did not exist for these families and is probably becoming an increasingly rare phenomenon. In common with kinship support, neighbourhood support has become less and less of a necessity as standards of living have risen, crises have become less frequent and the welfare state has provided a degree of protection against such crises as ill health and unemployment. However, perhaps the greatest single factor in the decline of close-knit neighbourhoods has been the large-scale re-housing that has taken place since the Second World War. The effect of slum clear-

ance and re-housing programmes has been to scatter existing neighbourhoods over large new housing estates and to create types of housing,
such as high rise flats, which are not conducive to the development of
neighbourhood relations. The nature of the housing combined with a
lack of local shopping centres, increased use of cars and more women
going out to work, has meant that the opportunities for neighbours to
meet each other have been sharply reduced.

What are the prospects for the future? There is no reason to suppose
that informal support networks will undergo a major revival. The basic
rationale for the existence of such networks on a day-to-day basis no
longer exists for the majority of families. The modern nuclear family
has a higher degree of independence because its needs are less and its
resources are greater. Kinship, friendship and neighbourhood networks
have become a matter of choice rather than necessity. Where supportive relationships do exist they tend to be more sporadic or to constitute
safety nets to be used in times of crisis rather than affecting day-to-day
family life.

The Services

The preceding discussion about the burden of care for the family, and
the present inadequacies of informal networks indicates that the
services must play an increasingly important part in the future in providing the support necessary to facilitate the severely mentally handicapped child remaining at home. How can services be developed to meet
more effectively the needs of families and ease the burdens presently
placed on mothers? The findings of this study justify a number of
practical recommendations which, if implemented, would result in a
marked improvement in the quality of life for large numbers of families
with severely mentally handicapped children. However, the structure
and general orientation of services and the knowledge and attitudes of
those responsible for providing them are equally important in determining their effectiveness in meeting the needs of families. The conclusions with regard to the various services that follow do not constitute
an attempt to provide an overall plan, but to suggest ways in which
some of the existing inadequacies which were highlighted in the study
might be overcome.

Education Services Whilst the principle concern of teachers and others
involved in the education of the mentally handicapped is, rightly, the
educational achievement of the child, it should be recognisedthat
relieving the burden on the family, and the mother in particular, is an

important secondary function. The concerns of this study caused it to focus on this secondary function rather than on the content of education, assessment procedures, learning programmes, etc.

The most widely felt need for additional support was for relief from twenty-four hours a day, seven days a week child care during the school holidays. At these times many mothers found the strain of coping with their handicapped child almost intolerable. Education authorities and social services departments working together should give the provision of day care during school holidays top priority. The buildings and equipment are already available in the special schools so that the cost of providing such care, during at least part of the school holidays, would not be too great when weighed against the benefits it would have for hard pressed mothers. It would, in addition, reduce the demand for short-term residential accommodation during the peak summer period. Initially, schemes to open schools during the holidays might only operate in certain areas, only cover part of the holidays and, in some cases, be staffed by volunteers, but the long-term objective should be to make this a statutory provision available in all areas and covering most of the school holidays.

Other times at which a high proportion of mothers wanted more help were at weekends and after normal school hours. The type of help that families wanted at weekends was rather different from that required in the school holidays. In most cases what was needed was someone to look after the handicapped child for two or three hours whilst parents spent time on other activities such as outings with their other children or shopping expeditions. This might be achieved by the establishment of voluntary playgroups, possibly making use of school facilities and possibly involving the parents themselves, or through the use of imaginative fostering arrangements where the foster family can be employed by the hour. The demand for care out of school hours came mostly from those mothers who wished to go out to work. It was less than the demand for care in the school holidays and would probably not justify the provision of a full-scale service for all families, but education authorities should consider the introduction of at least limited schemes to meet the needs of mothers who want to go out to work.

The recently published Warnock Report dealt with all aspects of special education for children with a wide variety of handicaps.[2] It included recommendations on making provisions for school holidays and on the possibility of extending school hours. It suggested that ways of enabling some special schools to remain open for at least part of the school holidays should be sought, although the committee rejected a general proposals for a four-term school year.[3] Similarly, it did not accept proposals for a general increase in the length of school hours in special schools, on the grounds that they should be kept broadly in line with ordinary schools. In both cases one can sympathise with the view that the lives of severely mentally handicapped children should be as much like those of other children as possible, but surely the normalisation of the lives of their parents should also be an objective. At present, these parents' prospects for employment, social and recreational activities are permanently restricted to an extent that parents of ordinary children only experience for a relatively short period of time. For these reasons there is a strong case for the opportunity to obtain extended school hours and care during the school holidays being made available to all parents of severely mentally handicapped children, although not all will wish to avail themselves of these services.

Two other problems which mothers frequently mentioned deserve to receive some attention from education authorities; arrangements for transporting children to and from school and the difficulties experienced in maintaining contact with teachers. Bussing arrangements were inevitably difficult, simply because the special school system meant that many children had to be brought considerable distances. In spite of this, however, there were ways in which transport arrangements might have been improved. If all schools had their own transport it should be possible to achieve more flexibility, e.g. it would be possible for children to stay on for club sessions after school. Also there is no reason why, with careful planning, the service could not be made more reliable. Finally, in some cases, alternative arrangements such as supervised travel on public transport or rota arrangements for families with cars might be possible. The problem of maintaining contact with teachers was also largely a consequence of the distance between home and school. There are a number of ways in which communication between home and school might be improved. First, and most important, the schools should encourage parents to visit at any time during the ordinary school day and teachers should be prepared to discuss with parents their children's learning programme and progress. Secondly, although most schools already have parents' evenings and open days, these might be made more accessible, e.g. the schools might be able to help with baby-sitting or transport problems which often prevent parents from attending. Thirdly, where parents have a telephone they should be encouraged to maintain contact with the school through this means and to discuss problems directly with the teachers. Finally, it might be a great help to both the teacher and the parents if the teacher were to visit the family at home to discuss the child's progress.

Health Services   The roles of the various health professions and specialists within the professions in the care of the mentally handicapped in the community have become very confused as a result of the many changes in structure and organisation that have taken place over the years. The experiences of families in this study with various health service personnel were extremely patchy, perhaps reflecting this confusion. The situation might be improved with the advent of the district handicap teams recommended in the Court Report on child health services.[4] Such teams will be multi-disciplinary, including representatives of social services departments, and will be responsible for all types of handicapped children within a health district (population around 200,000). These teams should provide an additional point of contact with the health services for families with a mentally handicapped child, through which they can have access to information, assessment, treatment and other services. However, the range of responsibilities of the district handicap team seems too wide for it to provide a satisfactory service. There is also a need for a community mental handicap team serving a much smaller population, with a specific responsibility for the mentally handicapped and an ability to liaise with both the district handicap team and the primary health care team (GPs, community nurses, health visitors, etc.). Such a community team would, like the district handicap team, be multi-disciplinary and a detailed outline of its function and composition has recently been elaborated in the first report of the National Development Team.[5] They envisage that such a team would have at its disposal the services of other professionals such as psychologists, speech therapists, etc., and the facilities of a community unit including short-term residential accommodation situated within easy reach of the families. The team would provide both a continuing service, where this was necessary, and a back-up to existing services which were either unable or unwilling to meet the needs of the family.

The two health service workers who are likely to have most contact with families on a day-to-day basis are the GP and the community nurse. Many GPs unfortunately show a marked lack of knowledge and understanding about the mentally handicapped. It is most important that all doctors have some basic knowledge of the severely mentally handicapped and the problems that families experience in caring for such individuals. In-service training courses might do something to remedy the existing situation, but the long-term solution must lie in more attention being paid to mental handicap in the medical curriculum, possibly at the expense of attention currently paid to more spectacular but less common conditions. The involvement of community nurses and health visitors with the mentally handicapped and their families varies enormously from one area to another. In some cases, families in the present study who required such essentials as incontinence aids were not receiving them, either because of a lack of contact with the community nursing service, or because of the difficulty of obtaining suitable aids. However, the role of the community nurse should extend far beyond the provision of incontinence aids. The gradual development of community mental handicap nursing as a specialty, often recruiting nurses from mental handicap hospitals who have long experience of working with the mentally handicapped, should produce a marked improvement in the service provided for families. The community mental handicap nurse can play a very important role by working directly with the family in their own home. He or she should be able to work with the parents in the development of self-help skills in the handicapped child, advise on problems of physical care such as how to lift a non-ambulant child and advise parents on the handling of behaviour problems. The Wessex Portage Scheme has already demonstrated the value of home-based teaching, particularly for the pre-school handicapped child.[6] Ideally, the role of the community nurse should complement rather than duplicate that of the social worker, although it is likely that where social work support is inadequate the nurse will find himself or herself providing the sort of help to families that would normally be the province of the social worker.

Nothing has so far been said about the mental handicap hospitals. Despite the intention to reduce gradually the size of the larger hospitals and to avoid the admission of children who do not require nursing care, it will be many years before they cease to play an important part. Their most important function for families caring for severely mentally handicapped children at home is in providing short-term accommodation. The provision of more local authority residential accommodation and possibly health service community units, should result in a decline in the importance of the hospitals in providing short-term care, but in the light of the heavy demand for short-term places this is likely to be a slow process. The Wessex Regional Health Authority has pioneered the introduction and evaluation of small hospital units for severely mentally handicapped children but most other authorities lag far behind.[7] In the meantime, conditions in many of the large hospitals, although they have improved considerably, still leave a great deal to be desired, and upgrading and improved staffing ratios are urgently required. In addition, steps should be taken to improve the access that parents have to the hospitals. Arrangements for the admission of children to short-term care should, as far as possible, take place between the parents and the hospital staff rather than through intermediaries. This should constitute part of a process of increasing the links between the hospitals and the communities they serve. This process has already affected the roles of consultants and nurses in mental handicap, and its further development should result in a marked improvement in the services that families receive from the hospitals.

Social Services   Social services departments have a vital role to play in meeting the needs of the severely mentally handicapped and their families and thus creating a system of community care which presents families with a viable alternative to seeking long-term care for the child. Unfortunately, most of them are not at present playing this role. In many areas the quality and quantity of support services available to families has not improved since the reorganisation of social services departments in 1971. There are many reasons for this, but two of the most important are, first, the wide ranging responsibilities of these departments, and second, the imposition of severe budgetary constraints. They are responsible for meeting the needs of such diverse groups as low-income families, mental patients in the community and mentally or physically infirm old people. The severely mentally handicapped constitute a very small part of their overall responsibilities and hence they are easily neglected in the face of rapidly increasing demands from other sections of the population. The financial constraints of the past four or five years have not made the task of the social services departments any easier. They are an obvious target for cuts in local authority spending designed to reduce the burden on the rates. Nevertheless, services to groups such as the severely mentally handicapped must be improved if the whole concept of community care is not to fall into disrepute.

   The role of the social worker is fundamental to the provision of effective support to families. One of the consequences of the reorganisation into social services departments was the gradual disappearance of the specialist social worker, to be replaced by the generic worker who was supposed to have a case load which reflected the wide variety of clients dealt with by the social services departments. In principle the idea had many advantages, in terms of integrating the work of the many diverse parts of the service. In practice it has led to a lack of specialised knowledge on the part of social workers, particularly in relation to relatively small client groups with special needs such as the mentally handicapped. The solution to this problem is not a simple return to the old ways, which were usually far from satisfactory. Social services departments should be seeking ways of introducing social workers who are specially trained to work with the mentally handicapped, but who would also work with generic teams. These individuals could take on the more difficult cases themselves, but at the same time they could serve an advisory and educative function in relation to other social workers who would retain some families on their own case loads. Such developments would, however, need to take place alongside a change in the sort of relationship that social workers have with families; from crisis management to long-term prevention. As long as social workers are only able to respond to immediate crises they will frequently find themselves unable to solve the long-term problems that families face, partly because the situation has gone too far and partly because they lack a close understanding of all the circumstances. Through long-term contact with the family, beginning as soon as the child is identified as severely mentally handicapped, the social worker could become aware of the needs of the family and the resources that they have at their disposal to meet these needs. The focus should be upon working with members of the family to seek practical solutions to practical problems, although there will be occasions on which emotional and psychological support is also necessary. The solutions to problems will often require the provision of supportive services, but the social worker should also discuss with family members how family and community resources might be better utilised. Thus, the father might be encouraged to participate more in the care of the handicapped child, or relatives may be asked to help with baby-sitting. In this way the impact that social workers have on the problems of families might be greatly increased.

An important aspect of the social workers' function is to provide access to a range of practical support services provided by social services departments and other agencies. The availability of these services is extremely patchy at present and some, although available in theory, are only rarely provided. A wide range of domiciliary services (e.g. home helps, laundry, telephone installations, the provision of aids, adaptations to housing, etc.) is provided for an equally wide range of client groups (e.g. the elderly, the physically handicapped, the mentally handicapped, etc.), but the results of the present study suggest that many families with mentally handicapped children who would benefit from the privision of such services are not receiving them. In particular, home helps and laundry services seem, in some areas, to be reserved almost exclusively for the elderly, although they were intended to serve other client groups as well. A reaffirmation from the DHSS that such services should be available to families with severely mentally handicapped children would be welcome, but it is also important that social workers should insist on certain families receiving this support. Not only is it necessary to ensure that existing services are provided, but it is also important that social services departments should consider the establishment of new services where these are necessary. In particular, large numbers of families would welcome help with baby-sitting and transport problems. The cost of providing a baby-sitting service might be relatively small, since such a service could involve both parents and volunteers. In the case of transport problems, the first priority is to ensure that families are receiving the mobility allowance, but it may also be necessary to seek ways of providing practical support with these problems.

The other major form of support which social services departments can provide, and which may in the long run have an important effect on the family's ability to cope with the handicapped child at home, is short-term residential accommodation. Many departments have failed to meet their obligation to provide residential facilities for severely mentally handicapped children who do not require hospital care, usually because of a lack of funds with which to build, equip and staff residential units. The problems of funding such projects will be briefly discussed later, but it is imperative that local authorities should do more to discharge their responsibilities in this area. Where residential units are opened they must include sufficient accommodation to meet the need for short-term care. Such units should be situated within the community that they serve and should establish a direct relationship with the families. Short-term care should not be seen solely as a means of providing relief during the school holidays. It can be used throughout the year to provide relief or just to enable the family to do things, such as going away for a weekend, which would otherwise be impossible. Some children might attend as weekly boarders and others might go for weekends. Such flexibility in arrangements would be far more likely to meet the needs of families and would also enable them to use the facilities to cope with the occasional domestic crises which affect all families. In addition to residential facilities, more authorities are now exploring the possibilities of short-term fostering of mentally handicapped children. In some areas imaginative schemes are already operating in which foster families negotiate directly with the parents of a mentally handicapped child, taking the child for periods ranging from a few hours to a week. Such schemes offer the advantages of flexibility combined with the opportunity for foster parents to develop a continuing relationship with the handicapped child.

Voluntary Agencies   There are many voluntary agencies which are concerned with the needs of the mentally handicapped, both providing direct support and acting as pressure groups seeking to improve statutory services. In terms of direct support to families, their activities range from organising parties and outings to providing short-term residential care. Whilst voluntary support cannot be a substitute for basic statutory provisions which families receive as of right, it does have a very important part to play. The government has begun to recognise the importance of the practical support that these groups provide by making substantial sums of money available to some to help them in their work. In many instances, the initiative to provide schemes such as play groups, summer holiday care provision and locally-based residential units has come from voluntary groups. Many of these schemes have the added advantage that they also involve the parents in the planning and running of them. It is important that voluntary groups should attempt to work in partnership with education, health and social services, but it is also important that they retain their independence, since they are the only alternative agencies to whom parents can turn. They are able to press the case for better services at national and local levels and to take up individual cases where the support families have received has been unsatisfactory.

What Sort of Services?   With specific reference to social workers, the point was made above that it was necessary to seek an alternative to services that seek only to manage short-term crises. Whilst there are considerable variations between services and between areas there is a general tendency to adopt the attitude that, as long as families are not complaining, then they must be coping adequately. If our objective is to devise services which will enable families to care for their handicapped children for as long as possible, then support must be provided long before they reach a point where they can no longer cope with the problems. It is obviously difficult for services with limited resources to devote some of these to families who are not apparently facing an immediate crisis,but unless this can be done there is little hope of preventing future crises which, in one way or another, the services will have to contend with at a later stage. In order to provide the sort of support necessary to prevent breakdown the services must be closely in touch with families and the everyday problems they experience. This applies equally to education, health and the social services. The needs and resources of families and individuals in families vary enormously. The problems faced by a family with an incontinent non-ambulant child who requires full physical care are very different from those faced by a family with a fully ambulant child with behaviour problems who does not require physical care. Only through close contact and the avail-ability of effective domiciliary services is it possible to identify and meet the needs of different families, and thus prevent crises which often lead to the decision to seek long-term care for the handicapped child. However, such an approach would require a degree of flexibilty and collaboration on the part of the various agencies which does not appear to exist at present.

Co-ordination and Collaboration   Fundamental to the development of the sorts of services that have been referred to here is a high degree of co-ordination and collaboration within and between various agencies. This should affect every level of planning and delivery of services. The National Development Group went so far as to say that: 'there should be no significant development of mental handicap services, whether on the side of the health authority or the local authority, unless planning has been undertaken on a joint basis'.[8] The establishment of joint care planning teams at local authority and area health authority level was suggested by the government in 1976. Most areas now have such teams and the establishment of sub-groups of joint care planning teams dealing specifically with services for the mentally handicapped is an important step forward, although in many areas these are still in their infancy. As well as planning services for the mentally handicapped, the exercise could be further extended to the preparation of joint information documents for parents on the range of services available to them and their handicapped children. A number of parents' organisations have prepared such pamphlets as have some of the more progressive social services departments, but it is important that all those involved in the delivery of the various services get together to produce joint publica-tions for their area.[9] The extension of collaboration to the actual delivery of services may prove more difficult, but it is nevertheless just as important. Professions such as community mental handicap nurses and social workers should be aware of each other's roles and have ready access to the services provided by other professions and other agencies. The community mental handicap teams proposed by the National Development Group and the National Development Team, if implemented, hold out the prospect of dramatic improvements in the degree of co-ordination and collaboration.

Accountability The variability in the quantity and quality of services provided in different areas and even in the same area has been mentioned many times in this book. What is a satisfactory standard of service and to whom should parents complain if they feel they or their children are not receiving satisfactory services? There are, as yet, no good answers to these questions. Standards of provision, other than certain basic minimum standards are not yet laid down and even where there is some guidance there is little the consumer can do if he or she feels a particular authority is failing to live up to these standards. The establishment of the community health councils constitutes a minimal start in this direction in that the parents now have somebody to complain to if they feel there are inadequacies in the health services. However, experience of the community health councils suggests that even they are variable, since their function seems to be ill-defined and open to a range of interpretations. To some extent voluntary bodies such as the National Society for Mentally Handicapped Children act as watchdogs in relation to the various stautory agencies, but the establishment of more formal machinery through which complaints can be made must be a top priority.

Who Pays? So far in this discussion, the problem of paying for these numerous improvements in services has not been raised, but many of the proposed improvements could be implemented for relatively little extra cost. More flexibility in school hours, the establishment of specialist teams, making home helps and laundry facilities available, etc. would not be major items of expenditure. An important initial step is to persuade authorities to look at those aspects of their services that might be improved at little extra cost. The excellent pamphlet from the National Development Group, 'Mentally Handicapped Children: A Plan for Action', provides authorities with a checklist of items, divided into those that can be achieved at relatively small cost and those that will involve more significant expenditure.[10] As far as more expensive projects, such as the provision of residential units is concerned, the National Development Group feels that improvements in mental handicap services in the coming years will depend, in large measure, on the extent to which joint financing can be brought to bear on service development. The government issued a circular on joint planning and joint financing in 1977 which stated that joint financing was 'designed to allow the limited and controlled use of resources available to health authorities for the purposes of support in selected personal social services spending by local authorities'.[11] This money can be used for both capital and revenue expenditure for the mentally handicapped as well as for other groups. It can be used to protect services threatened by expenditure cuts and also to develop new projects. Local authorities should be given every encouragement to make use of this money to improve services in their areas. Nevertheless, the view that services should not be greatly affected by the shortage of resources is perhaps somewhat optimistic. The sort of improvements that are necessary in education, community health services and domiciliary social services do require considerable additional resources and no proposals for the implementation of these improvements can be considered outside of the wider economic and political context.

The Economic and Political Context

Expenditure on services for the severely mentally handicapped and their families is a small part of total state expenditure in Britain. State expenditure as a whole has expanded rapidly during this century. From a level of around 15 per cent of gross national product before the First World War it rose to 30 per cent in the inter-war period and achieved a level of over 50 per cent of gross national product by the late 1960s. On the other hand, the past 30 years have seen a decline in the British economy relative to the economies of other advanced industrial societies. The fact that much state expenditure is devoted to non-productive uses has been identified by many political and economic commentators as a major reason for current economic problems. They have argued that expenditure on health and social services must be constrained in order to promote expemditure on investment in industrial production, although, in fact, Britain lags behind most Western European countries in the proportion of GNP devoted to health and social services. It has been against this background that the policy of community care has become popular among politicians in recent years. It has been advocated on humanitarian grounds and because it is hoped that it will provide an opportunity to reduce the cost of providing care, it is supposedly better and cheaper than the alternatives. In practice, for some client groups, the policy of community care has merely provided moral justification for reductions in the services. So far, the mentally handicapped and their families have suffered perhaps less than other groups because their previous history of neglect provided little scope for reductions in expenditure. The danger of attempting to pursue a policy of community care without providing the resources necessary to improve community services is that an increasingly heavy burden will be placed on the mothers of the mentally handicapped, many of whom, as we have seen, are already carrying an almost intolerable burden of care. Community care can only be acceptable and can only work if it means more support available to more families, and this in turn means that more resources will have to be devoted to providing this support. The solution to current economic problems will never be found in resorting to attacks on the weakest sections of the population.

NOTES

CHAPTER 1

1. M. Adams, *Mental Retardation and its Social Domensions* (Columbia University Press, New York, 1971), p. 1.

2. R. Pushkin, 'Community confusion over abnormality needs: a remedy', *Health and Social Services Journal* 15 Oct. 1976, 1856-7.

3. M. Adams, *Mental Retardation*, p. 2.

4. J.R. Mercer, 'The meaning of mental retardation', in R. Koch & J.C. Dobson (eds), *The Mentally Retarded Child and his Family* (Brunner Mazell, New York, 1971), p. 27.

5. For an excellent description of the attempts of people classified as mentally retarded to pass as normal see R.B. Edgerton, *The Cloak of Competence: Stigma in the Lives of the Mentally Retarded* (University of California Press, Berkley, 1967).

6. Quoted in J.R. Mercer, 'The meaning of mental retardation', p. 2 6.

7. K. Soddy, 'The clinical picture', in M. Adams and H. Lovejoy, (London, Heineman, 1972), p. 20.

8. M. Mannoni, *The Child, His Illness and Others* (Tavistock, London, 1970).

9. R.B. Edgerton *The Cloak of Competence*.

10. A. Kushlick and R. Blunden 'The epidemiology of mental subnormality', in A.M. Clarke and A.D.B. Clarke, *Mental Deficiency: The Changing Outlook* (Methuen, London, 1974).

11. DHSS, *Better Services for the Mentally Handicapped* (HMSO, London, 1971), Cmnd. 4683, p. 1.

12. T. Fryers 'Severe mental handicap: The dynamics of prevalence: Epidemiology in an English city 1961-77', unpublished PhD Thesis (University of Manchester, 1978).

13. A.M. Clarke and A.D.B. Clarke, *Mental Deficiency*, p. 16.

14. K. Jones, *A History of the Mental Health Services* (Routledge & Kegan Paul, London, 1972).

15. Ibid., pp. 182-3.

16. Quoted in A.M. Clarke and A.D.B. Clarke, *Mental Deficiency*, p. 17.

17. K. Jones *History of the Mental Health Services*, p. 208.

18. W.B. Jaehnig, 'The Mentally handicapped and their families', unpublished P Thesis (University of Essex, 1974).

19. B. Hollander, *Abnormal Children* (Kegan Paul Trench Trubner & Co. London, 1913), p. 39.

20. K. Jones, *History of the Mental Health Services*, p. 213.

21. F.C. Shrubshall and A.C. Williams, *Mental Deficiency Practice* (University of London Press, London, 1932), p. 161.

22. J. Bowlby, *Maternal Care and Mental Health* WHO, Geneva, 1952).

23. R. Titmuss, 'Community care: Fact or fiction', in R. Titmuss, *Commitment to Welfare* (Unwin, London, 1961), pp. 104-5.

24. Ministry of Health *Health and Welfare: The Development of Community Care* (HMSO, London, 1963), Cmnd. 1973.

25. Ibid., p. 25.

26. P. Mittler, 'The Mental Health Services', *Fabian Research Series*, 252 (1966), p. 12.

27. *Report of the Committee on Local Authority and Allied Social Services*

(HMSO, London, 1968), Cmnd. 3703.

28. W.B. Jaehnig, 'Domiciliary services for the mentally handicapped – Beyond community care', in *The Mentally Handicapped: An Effectivē Service*, Proceedings of a conference, Campaign for the Mentally Handicapped and Dr Barnodos (1972), p. 72.

29. *Report of the Committee of Inquiry into Allegations of Ill-treatment of Patients and Other Irregularities at the Ely Hospital, Cardiff* (HMSO, London, 1969), Cmnd. 3795; *Report of the Farleigh Hospital Committee of Inquiry* (HMSO, London, 1971), Cmnd. 4557.

30. P. Morris, *Put Away: A Sociological Study of Institutions for the Mentally Retarded* (Routledge & Kegan Paul, London, 1969).

31. DHSS, *Better Services for the Mentally Handicapped*.

32. Ibid., p. 9.

33. Ibid., p. 42.

34. Text of Secretary of State's speech to the National Society for Mentally Handicapped Children Conference on Mental Handicap – Development of Resources, Feb. 1975.

35. K. Jones, *Opening the Door: A Study of New Policies for the Mentally Handicapped* (Routledge & Kegan Paul, London, 1975).

36. Ibid.

37. J. Newson and E. Newson, 'Foreword' to S. Hewett, *The Need for Long Term Care*, Inst. for Res. into Ment. Retard.Occ. Papers No. 3 (Butterworth, London, 1972).

38. Ibid., p. 61.

39. B. Spain and G. Wigley (eds), *Right from the Start: A Service for Families with a Young Handicapped Child* (HNMHC, London,1975); Campaign for the Mentally Handicapped, *Even Better Services for the Mentally Handicapped* (1972 (1972), Kings Fund Centre, *Services for Mentally Handicapped Children* (Kings Fund, London, 1976); British Association of Social Workers, *Better Services for the Mentally Handicapped: Report of the Working Party on the White Paper* (BASW, Birmingham, undated).

40. National Development Group for the Mentally Handicapped, *Mentally Handicapped Children: A Plan for Action*, Pamphlet No. 2 (National Development Group for the Mentally Handicapped, London, 1976); National Development Group for the Mentally Handicapped, *Helping Mentally Handicapped School Leavers*, Pamphlet No. 3 (National Development Group for the Mentally Handicapped, London, 1977); National Development Group for the Mentally Handicapped *Day Services for Mentally Handicapped Adults*, Pamphlet No. 5 (National Development Group for the Mentally Handicapped, London 1977).

41. Report of the Committee on Child Health Services, *Fit for the Future* (HMSO, London, 1976); Report of the Committee of Enquiry into the Education of Handicapped Children and Young People, *Special Educational Needs* (HMSO, London, 1978).

CHAPTER 2

1. Bowlby, Maternal Care and Mental Health (WHO, Geneva, 1952).

2. Tizard, J. 'The residential care of mentally handicapped children', in B.W. Richards (ed.), *Proceedings of the London Conference of the Association for the Scientific Study of Mental Deficiency* (May & Baker, Dagenham, 1960); J.G. Lyle 'The effect of an institutional upon the verbal development of imbecile children III: The Brooklands residential family unit', *J. Ment. Res.* 4 (1960) 14-23; S.A. Centrewall and W.A. Centrewall, 'A study of children with mongolism reared in the home compared to those reared away from home', *Paediatrics*, 25 (1960)

212 *Notes*

678-85.

3. A. Dupont 'Severely mentally retarded children at home', *REAP*, 1 (nov. 1975) 107-12.

4. S. Kew, *Handicap and Family Crisis* (Pitman, London, 1975).

5. S. Hewett, *The Family and the Handicapped Child* (George Allen & Unwin, London, 1970); W.B. Jaehnig, 'Mentally handicapped children and their families: Problems for social policy', unpublished PhD Thesis (University of Essex).

6. Ibid. pp. 31-2.

7. S. Hewett, *The Family and the Handicapped Child*, p. 194.

8. W.B. Jaenhig, 'Mentally handicapped children', p. 311.

9. M. Voysey, *A Constant Burden: The Reconstitution of Family Life* (Routledge & Kegan Paul, London, 1975).

10. M. Adams and H. Lovejoy, *The Mentally Subnormal: Social Work Approaches* (Heinemann, London, 1972), p. 80.

11. W.B. Jaehnig, 'Mentally handicapped children', p. 179.

12. K.S. Holt, 'The home care of the severely mentally retarded', *Paediatrics*, 22 (1958) 744-55.

13. W.B. Jaehnig, 'Mentally handicapped children',

14. A.I. Roth 'The myth of parental attitudes', *Journal of Mental Subnormality*, 9 (1963) 51-4.

15. Examples of studies using third party evaluations are: L.C. Wolf and P.C. Whitehead, 'The decision to institutionalise retarded children: A comparison of individually matched groups', *Mental Retardation*, 13 (1975) 3-7; S. Kew, *Handicap and Family Crisis*; examples of studies using assessment through psychological questionnaires are: S.T. Cummings, H.C. Bailey, H.E. Rie,'Effects of the child's deficiency on the mother: A study of mothers of mentally retarded, chronically ill and neurotic children', *American Journal of Orthopsychiatry*, 36 (1966) 595-609; J.R. Peck and W.B. Stephens 'A study of the relationship between the attitudes and behaviour of parents and that of their mentally defective child', *American Journal of Mental Deficiency*, 74 (1960) 839-43.

16. J.K. McMichael, *Handicap: A Study of Physically Handicapped Children and their Families* (Staples, London, 1971).

17. R. Mackieth, 'The feelings and behaviour of parents of handicapped children', *Developmental Medicine and Child Neurology*, 15 (1973) 524-7.

18. W. Wolfensberger, 'Counselling parents of the retarded', in A. Baumeister (ed.), *Mental Retardation* (University of London Press, London., 1967).

19. A. Gath, *Down's Syndrome and the Family* (Academic Press, London, 1978), p. 116.

20. L. Wing, 'Problems experienced by parents of children with severe mental retardation', in B. Spain and G. Wigley *Right from the Start*; E.H. Hare and G.K. Shaw, *Mental Health on a New Housing Estate* (Oxford University Press, London, 1965); M. Shepherd, A.C. Brown and G.W. Kalton, *Psychiatric Illness in General Practice* (Oxford University Press, London, 1966).

21. B. Farber, 'Effects of a severely mentally retarded child on family integration', *Monograph of Social Research in Child Development*, No. 71 (1959), M. Fowle, 'The effect of the severely mentally retarded child on his family', *American Journal of Mental Deficiency*, 13 (1959) 468.

22. S. Kew, *Handicap and Family Crisis*.

23. E.K. Grossman, *Brothers and Sisters of Retarded Children* (Syracuse University Press, New York, 1972).

24. B. Farber, 'Effects of a severely mentally retarded child'.

25. J. Carr, 'The effect of the severely mentally subnormal on their families', in A.M. Clarke and A.D.B. Clarke, *Mental Deficiency: The Changing Outlook*

26. J. Tizard and J.C. Grad, *Mentally Handicapped Children and their Families* (Oxford University Press, London, 1961).

27. M. Fowle, 'The effect of the severely mentally retarded child'.
28. S. Schild, 'The family of the retarded child', in R. Koch and J.C. Dobson (eds), *The Mentally Retarded Child and His Family* (Brunner Mazel, New York, 1971).
29. B. Farber, 'Perceptions of crisis related variables in the impact of the retarded child on the mother', *Journal of Health and Human Behaviour*, 1 (1960) 108-18.
30. B. Farber, *Mental Handicap: Its Social Context and Social Consequences* (Houghton Mifflin, Boston, 1968).
31. K.S. Holt, 'Home care'.
32. S. Hewett, *The Family and the Handicapped Child*, p. 121.
33. For a discussion of the problems of presenting handicap to outsiders see: R.H. Barsch, 'Explanations offered by parents and siblings of brain injured children', *Exceptional Children*, 27 (1961) 286-91; W.B. Jaehnig 'Mentally handicapped children'; M. Voysey, *A Constant Burden*.
34. J. Carr, 'Effects on the family of a child with Down's Syndrome', *Physiotherapy*, 62 (1976) 20-4.
35. M. Culver, 'Intergenerational social mobility among families with a severely mentally retarded child', unpublished PhD dissertation (University of Illinois, 1967). Quoted in B. Farber, *Mental Handicap*, p. 163.
36. S. Lloyd-Bostock, 'Parents, experiences of official help and guidance in caring for a mentally handicapped child', *Child Care Health Development*, 2 (1976) 325-38.
37. S. Hewett, *The Family and the Handicapped Child*; M. Bayley, *Mental Handicap and Community Care* (Routledge & Kegan Paul, London, 1973); W.B. Jaehnig 'Mentally handicapped children'; J. Carr, 'Effects on the family'.
38. S. Hewett, ibid.
39. J. Carr, 'Effects on the family'.
40. See M. Bayley, *Mental Handicap and Community Care*.
41. W.B. Jaehnig 'The mentally handicapped and their families', unpublished Research Report (University of Essex, 1973), pp. 28-30.
42. J. Tizard and J.C. Grad, *Mentally Handicapped Children* pp. 56-63.
43. J. Moncrieff, *Mental Subnormality in London: A Survey of Community Care* (PEP, London, 1966).
44. W.B. Jaehnig, 'Mentally handicapped and their families', pp. 34-41.
45. J. Carr, 'Effect of the severely mentally subnormal'.
46. A.R. Schaffer, 'The too-cohesive family: A form of group pathology', *Social Psychiatry*, vol. X, no. 4 (1964).
47. S. Hewett, *The Family and the Handicapped Child*, p. 107.
48. J. Carr, 'Effects on the family'.
49. M. Bayley, *Mental Handicap and Community Care*, p. 265.
50. Ibid., pp. 267-70.
51. Ibid., pp. 342-4.
52. J. Tizard, 'Services and evaluation of services', in A.M. Clarke and A.D.B. Clarke, *Mental Deficiency*, p. 848.
53. M. Bayley, *Mental Handicap and Community Care*; W.B. Jaehnig 'Mentally handicapped children'; C. Glendenning, 'The handicapped child in the community', (University of York, Department of Social Administration and Social Work, 1978); A.M. Fox, 'They get this training but they don't really know how you feel', *Action Research for the Crippled Child* (1974); M. McCormack, *A Mentally Handicapped Child in the Family* (Constable, London, 1978).
54. M. Bayley, *Mental Handicap and Community Care*, p. 309.
55. W.B. Jaehnig, 'Mentally handicapped children', p. 314.
56. D. Hitch, 'What help can parents get? A family fund analysis', *Concern*, 23 (Spring, 1977) 6-12.

57. L. Wing, 'Severely retarded children in a London area: Prevalence and provision of services', *Psychological Medicine*, 1 (1971) 405-15.

58. C.G. Schwartz, 'Strategies and tactics of mothers of mentally retarded children for dealing with the medical care system', in N. Bernstein (ed.), *Diminished People: The Problems and Care of the Mentally Retarded* (Little Brown, Boston, 1970).

59. W.B. Jaehnig, 'Mentally handicapped children', p. 20.

60. L. Wing, 'Practical counselling for families, with severely mentally retarded children living at home', *REAP* (Nov. 1975) 113-17.

61. Hewett found that, when mothers were asked whom they would turn to if they needed help, 35 per cent named voluntary organisations. S. Hewett, *The Family and the Handicapped Child*, pp. 170-1.

62. E. Younghusband, D. Birchall, R. Davie and M.L. Kellmer Pringle, *Living with Handicap* (National Children's Bureau, (London, 1970), p. 95.

63. J. Tizard and J.C. Grad, *Mentally Handicapped Children*; J. Leeson, 'A study of six young mentally handicapped children and their families', *The Medical Officer*, 104 (1960) 331-14.

64. DHSS, *Better Services for the Mentally Handicapped* (HMSO, London, 1971), Cmnd. 4683, p. 10.

65. M. Bayley, *Mental Handicap and Community Care*, p. 12.

66. Ibid., p. 297.

67. W.B. Jaehnig, 'Mentally handicapped children', p. 259.

68. J. Carr, 'Effects on the family'.

69. L. Burton, *The Family Life of Sick Children: A study of Families Coping with Chronic Childhood Disease* (Routledge & Kegan Paul, London, 1975), p. 123.

70. DHSS, *Better Servcices*, p. 43.

71. P. Morris, *Put Away: A Sociological Study of Institutions; Report of the Farleigh Hospital Committee of Inquiry* (HMSO, London, 19 , Cmnd. 4557; *Report of the Committee of Inquiry into Allegations of Ill-Treatment of Patients and other Irregularities at the Ely Hospital, Cardiff*.

72. J. Tizard and J.C. Grad, *Mentallv Handicapped Children*, p. 21; G. Saenger, 'Factors influencing the institutionalisation of mentally retarded individuals in New York City', *American Sociological Review* (1960); B.V. Graliker, R. Koch and R.A. Henderson, 'Factors influencing placement of retarded children in a state residential institution', *American Journal of Mental Deficiency*, 69 (1965) 553; J.R. Kershner, 'Intellectual and social development in relation to family functioning: A longitudinal comparison of home versus institutional effects', *American Journal of Mental Deficiency*, (1970) 75 276-84; D.N. Mackay and R. Elliot, 'Subnormals under hospital and community care', *Journal of Deficiency Research*, 19 (1975) 21-8.

73. G. Saenger, 'Factors influencing the institutionalisation'.

74. M.T. Hobbs, 'A comparison of institutionalised and non-institutionalised mentally retarded', *American Journal of Mental Deficiency*, 69 (1964) 206-10.

75. I. Tallman, 'Spousal role differentiation and the socialisation of severely retarded children', *Journal of Marriage and the Family*, 27 (1965) 37.

76. J. Tizard and J.C. Grad, *Mentally Handicapped Children*, p. 20; M. Bayley, *Mental Handicap and Community Care*, pp. 44-5; D.N. Mackay and R. Elliot, 'Subnormals under hospital and community care'.

77. D.N. Mackay and R. Elliot, 'Subnormals under hospital and community care'.

78. B.D. Singer and R. Osborn, 'Social class and sex differences in admission patterns of the mentally retarded', *American Journal of Mental Deficiency*, 75 (1970) 160-62; R.W. Olsen, 'Sex differences among hospital admissions: Fact or artifact', *Mental Retardation*, 5 (1967) 6-9.

79. Graliker *et al.*, 'Factors influencing placement'; W.B. Jaehnig, 'The mentally handicapped and their families', pp. 51-2.

80. J. Moncrieff, *Mental Subnormality in Families*, p. 29.

81. B. Farber, W.C. Jenne and R. Toigo, 'Family crisis and the decision to institutionalise the retarded child', Council for Exceptional Children, *NEA Research Mongraph Series No. A1* (1960); B. Farber and D.B. Ryckman, 'Effects of severely mentally retarded children on family relationships', *Mental Retardation Abstracts*, 2 (1965) 1-17.

82. S. Hewett, *The Need for Long Term Care*, Institute for Research into Mental Retardation, Occasional Papers, No. 3 (Butterworth, London, 1972).

83. M. Bayley, *Mental Handicap and Community Care*, pp. 87-90; W.B. Jaehnig, 'The mentally handicapped and their families' pp. 33-41.

84. S. Hewett, *Need for Long Term Care*.

85. M. Bayley, *Mental Handicap and Community Care*, p. 111.

86. J. Tizard and J.C. Grad, *Mentally Handicapped Children*; G. Saenger, 'Factors influencing the institutionalisation'; S. Hewett, *Need for Long Term Care*; M. Bayley, *Mental Handicap and Community Care*; W.B. Jaehnig, 'The mentally handicapped and their families'.

87. L.C. Wolf and P.C. Whitehead, 'The decision to institutionalise retarded children: A comparison of individually matched groups', *Mental Retardation*, 13 (1975) 3-7.

88. Ibid.

89. S. Hewett, *Need for Long Term Care*.

90. M. Bayley, *Mental Handicap and Community Care*, pp. 107-10.

91. S. Hewett, *Need for Long Term Care*.

92. W.B. Jaehnig, 'The mentally handicapped and their families'.

93. G. Saenger, 'Factors influencing the institutionalisation'.

94. M. Bone, B. Spain and F.M. Martin, Plans and Provisions for the Mentally Handicapped (Allen and Unwin, London, 1972).

95. M. Bayley, *Mental Handicap and Community Care*, p. 166.

96. W.B. Jaehnig 'The mentally handicapped and their families', pp. 400-1.

97. M. Bayley, *Mental Handicap and Community Care*, p. 165.

98. W.B. Jaehnig, 'The mentally handicapped and their families', p. 348.

CHAPTER 3

1. N. Dennis, F. Henriques and C. Slaughter, *Coal is Our Life* (Eyre and Spottiswoode, London, 1956). Quoted in A. Oakley, *Housewife* (Penguin, Harmondsworth, 1974).

2. R. Fletcher, *The Family and Marriage* (Penguin, Harmandsworth, 1962); R.O. Blood and D.M. Wolfe, *Husbands and Wives* (Free Press, New York, 1960); M. Young and P. Willmott, *The Symmetrical Family* (Routledge & Kegan Paul, London, 1973).

3. M. Young and P. Willmott, ibid.; Penguin edition (1975) p. 114.

4. E. Bott, *Family and Social Networks* (Tavistock, London, 1957).

5. B.E. Harrell-Bond, 'Conjugal role behaviour', *Human Relations*, 22 (1969) 77-91; J. Platt, 'Some problems in measuring the jointness of conjugal role relationships', *Sociology*, 3 (1969) 291. D.N. Toomey, 'Conjugal roles and social networks in an urban working class sample', *Human Relations*, 24 (1971) 417-31.

6. A. Oakley, *The Sociology of Housework* (Martin Robertson, London, 1974), p. 137.

7. M. Young and P. Willmott, *Symmetrical Family*, Penguin edition (1975) p. 115.

8. T. Parsons, 'The kinship system of the contemporary United States',

reprinted in T. Parsons, *Essays in Sociological Theory*, revised edition (Free Press, New York, 1964); For a comprehensive discussion of these questions see: D.H.J. Morgan, *Social Theory and the Family* (Routledge & Kegan Paul, London, 1975).

9. P. Laslett, *The World We Have Lost* (Methuen, London, 1965).

10. M. Anderson, *Family Structure in Nineteenth Century Lancashire* (Cambridge, CUP, 1971).

11. M. Young and P. Willmott, *Family and Kinship in East London* (Routledge & Kegan Paul, London, 1957).

12. P. Townsend, *The Family Life of Old People* (Routledge & Kegan Paul, London, 1957).

13. E. Litwak, 'Extended kin in an industrial society', in 'E. Shanas and G.F. Streib, *Social Structure and the Family: Generational Relations* (Prentice Hall, Englewood Clifs, 1965); M.B. Sussman and L. Burchenall, 'Kin family network: Unheralded structure in current conceptualisations of family functioning', in J.N. Edwards, *The Family and Change* (Knopf, New York, 1969).

14. C. Bull, *Middle Class Families* (Routledge & Kegan Paul, London, 1968).

15. E. Litwak and I. Szelenyi, 'Primary group structures and their functions: kin, neighbours and friends', *American Sociological Review* 34 (1969) 465-81. Excerpt in: M. Anderson, *Sociology of the Family* (Penguin, Harmondsworth, 1971).

16. E. Bott, 'Family and crisis', in J.S. Sutherland, *Towards Community Mental Health* (Tavistock, London, 1971).

17. M. Bayley, *Mental Handicap and Community Care*.

18. R. Plant, *Community and Ideology* (Routledge & Kegan Paul, London, 1974).

19. F. Tonnies, *Community and Association* (1887) reprinted (Routledge & Kegan Paul, London, 1955).

20. R. Plant, *Community and Ideology*, p. 13.

21. K.M. Webber, 'Towards a definition of the interest community', in P. Worlsey *et al.* (eds), *Modern Sociology* (Penguin, Harmondsworth, 1970).

22. D.W. Minor and S. Greer, (eds), *The Concept of Community* (Aldine Chicago, 1969).

23. Quoted in R. Titmuss, *Commitment to Welfare* (George Allen & Unwin, London, 1968).

24. *Report of the Committee on Local Authority and Allied Personal Social Services* (HMSO, London, 1968), Cmnd. 3703.

25. A. Forder, *Concepts in Social Administration* (Routledge & Kegan Paul, London, 1974).

26. J.E. Mayer and N. Timms, *The Client Speaks* (Routledge & Kegan Paul, London, 1970) p. 140.

27. MRC Social Psychiatry Unit *Schedule of Children's Handicaps, Behaviour and Skills* (1971).

28. H.C. Gunzberg, *Progress Assessment Charts* (National Association for Mental Health, London, 1966); E.A. Doll, The Vineland Social Maturity Scale: Manual of Directions (Educational Test Bureau, Minneapolis, 1947).

CHAPTER 4

1. B.D. Singer and R. Osborn, 'Social class and sex differences in admission patterns of the mentally retarded', *American Journal of Mental Deficiency*, 75 (1970) 16002; R.W. Olsen, 'Sex differences among hospital admissions: Fact or artefact', *Mental Retardation*, 5 (1967) 6-9.

2. T. Fryers, 'Severe mental handicap: The dynamics of prevalence: Epidemiology in an English city 1961-77', unpublished PhD Thesis (University of

Manchester, 1978).

3. E.A. Doll, *The Vineland Social Maturity Scale: Manual of Directions.*

4. G.W. Brown and T. Harris, *Social Origins of Depression: A Study of Psychiatric Disorder in Women* (Tavistock, London, 1978).

5. S. Hewett, *The Need for Long Term Care*; W.B. Jaehnig, 'Mentally handicapped children and their families'.

6. J. Tizard and J.C. Grad, *Mentally Handicapped Children and their Families*; W.G. Jaehnig, 'The mentally handicapped and their families'.

7. K. Dunnell and A. Cartwright, *Medicine Takers, Prescribers and Hoarders* (Routledge & Kegan Paul, London, 1972), p. 20.

8. J. Tizard and J.C. Grad, *Mentally Handicapped Children*, pp. 56-63; M. Bayley, *Mental Handicap and Community Care* pp.87-90; W.B. Jaehnig 'Mentally handicapped children', pp. 33-41.

CHAPTER 6

1. A. Oakley, *Sociology of Housework.*

2. M. Young and P. Willmott, *The Symmetrical Family.*

3. A. Oakley, *Sociology of Housework*, p. 137.

4. Ibid., p. 139.

5. E. Bott, *Family and Social Networks* (Tavistock, London, 1957); H. Gavron, *The Captive Wife* (Routledge & Kegan Paul, London, 1966).

6. A. Oakley, *Sociology of Housework.*

7. *Ibid.;* J. Newson and E. Newson, *Infant Care in an Urban Community* (Allen and Unwin, London, 1963).

8. A. Oakley, *Sociology of Housework.*

9. DHSS, *Better Services for the Mentally Handicapped* (HMSO, London, 1971), Cmnd. 4683.

10. M. Young and P. Willmott, *Family and Kinship in East London.*

11. M. Bayley, *Mental Handicap and Community Care* p. 265; S. Hewett, *The Family and the Handicapped Child.*

12. W.B. Jaehnig, 'The mentally handicapped and their families', pp. 330-6.

13. M. Bayley, *Mental Handicap and Community Care*, pp. 270-4; J. Carr, 'Effects on the family of a child with Down's Syndrome', Physiotherapy, 62 (1976) 20-24.

14. S. Hewett, *The Family and the Handicapped Child*, p. 107.

15. A. Oakley, *Sociology of Housework*, p. 137.

CHAPTER 7

1. R.M. Titmuss, 'Community care: Fact or fiction', in R.M. Titmus, *Commitment to Welfare* (Allen and Unwin, London 1961).

2. *Report of the Committee of Enquriy into the Education of Handicapped Children and Young People* Cmnd. 7212. (HMSO, London, 1978),

3. J. Tizard and J.C. Grad, *The Mentally Handicapped and their Families*, pp. 94-113; W.B. Jaehnig, 'The mentally handicapped and their families'.

4. J. Tizard and J.C. Grad, *Mentally Handicapped and their families*, pp. 94-113.

5. Ibid., p. 109.

6. Ibid., p. 109.

7. S. Hewett, *The Family and the Handicapped Child* (George Allen and Unwin, London, 1970); M. Bayley, *Mental Handicap and Community Care;* W.B. Jaehnig, 'Mentally handicapped and their families'.

CHAPTER 8

1. M. Susser and W. Watson, *Sociology in Medicine* (Oxford University Press, London, 1962).

CHAPTER 9

1. M. Young and P. Willmott, *Family and Kinship in East London;*
P. Townsend, *The Family Life of Old People*; C. Bell, *Middle Class Families* (Routledge & Kegan Paul, London, 1968).

2. *Report of the Committee of Enquiry into the Education of Handicapped Children and Young People* (HMSO, London, 1978), Cmnd. 7212.

3. Ibid., pp. 161-2.

4. *Report of the Committee on Child Health Services. Fit for the Future* (HMSO, London, 1976).

5. National Development Team for the Mentally Handicapped, *First Report: 19776-77* (HMSO, London, 1978).

6. J. Smith, A. Kushlick, C. Glossop, *The Wessex Portage Project: A home teaching service for families with a pre-school mentqlly handicapped child* (Wessex Health Care Evaluation Research Team, Winchester, 1977), Part 1 of the Research Report no. 125.

7. D. Felce, A. Kushlick, B. Lunt and E. Powell, *Evaluation of Locally Based Hospital Units for the Mentally Handicapped in Wessex: detailed rules for the setting up and maintenance of the units* (Eessex Health Care Evaluation Research Team, Winchester, 1977), Research Report no. 124.

8. National Development Group for the Mentally Handicapped, 'Mental Handicap: Planning Together', Pamphlet No. 1 (National Development Group for the Mentally Handicapped, London, 1976).

9. In some areas local groups of the NSMHC have produced their own guides and Social Services Departments have sometimes produced guides but there has been no systematic attempt over the country as a whole to prepare guides to all services.

10. National Development Group for the Mentally Handicapped, 'Mentally Handicapped Children: A Plan for Action', Pamphlet No. 2 (National Development Group for the Mentally Handicapped, London, 1977).

11. DHSS *Joint Planning and Joint Financing, HC 77/17* (HMSO, London, 1977).

INDEX

Adams, M. 11n1, 33
admissions group: definition 74, 75; representativeness of samples 75, 76; response rate 76, 77
age of handicapped child: factor associated with admission 51, 81, 82; matching of samples 82, 93
American Association for Mental Deficiency 13
Anderson, M. 64

baby sitting: fathers 127; level of support 115; mothers' needs for support 175, 186, 204; relatives 141; siblings 136, 137
Bayley, M. 40, 44-6, 48, 53, 54, 100, 145
behaviour problems: definition 89; effect of age 91, 92; effect on felt needs of mothers 180; factor associated with admission 50, 89-92; in public places 91; in school 150
Bell, C. 67
Better Services for the Mentally Handicapped (White Paper) 16, 24, 25, 27, 43, 48, 49, 139, 148
Birchenall, L. 65
birth order of handicapped child 51, 52
Blood, R.O. 61n2
Blunden, R. 16n10
Bone, M. 54n94
Bott, E. 62, 66, 129
Bowlby, E.J.M. 21, 30
British Association of Social Workers 27n39
brothers and sisters *see* siblings
Brown, G.W. 96
Burton, L. 48n69

Campaign for the Mentally Handicapped 27n39
Carr, J. 37, 40, 42, 44, 48, 145
Cartwright, A. 100
Castle, B. 27
Centrewall, S.A. 30n2
Centrewall, W. 30n2
child guidance 21

Chronically Sick and Disabled Persons Act 26
Clarke, A.D.B. 17n13
Clarke, A.M. 17n13
community 28, 57, 67-9, 73, 79, 93, 118, 139
community care 144, 147, 185; Better Services for the Mentally Handicapped 24, 139; cost 27, 207, 208; economic and political factors 20, 27, 208; effects of social change 28, 196; formal support 45-7; *in* or *by* the community 45, 146; informal support 28, 47-9, 55, 66, 67, 195-7; meaning of 43, 56-8, 123, 189, 190; Mental Health Act, 1959 21, 22; Seebohm Report 23; Wood Committee 20, *see also* family care
Community Health Councils 207
Constant Attendance Allowance 26, 42, 46, 103, 147
consumer durables 103, 104, *see also* standard of living
continence/incontinence 40, 84-6, 113, 155, 201
Court Report (Fit for the Future) 27n41, 200
Culver, M. 40n35
Cummings, S.T. 35n15

Dennis, N. 60n1
Department of Health and Social Security Census of Mental Handicap Patients in Hospitals (1972) 14, 15
Development Team for the Mentally Handicapped 200, 207
doctors: changing role in care of mentally handicapped 18-21; mental handicap specialists 156; mothers' comments 157; paediatricians 156; reaction to mothers' health problems 95, 96, *see also* general practitioners
Doll, E.A. 78n28
domestic routine: child minding 114-18; definitions of participation

219

For Product Safety Concerns and Information please contact our EU
representative GPSR@taylorandfrancis.com Taylor & Francis Verlag GmbH,
Kaufingerstraße 24, 80331 München, Germany

Printed and bound by CPI Group (UK) Ltd, Croydon, CR0 4YY
08/06/2025
01896991-0004